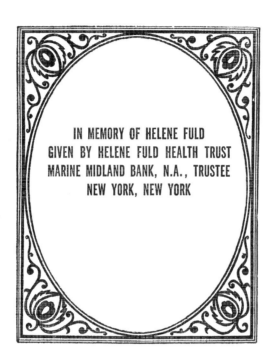

Photographic Anatomy of the Human Body

CHIHIRO YOKOCHI, M.D.
Professor, Department of Anatomy
Kanagawa Dental College
Yokosuka, Japan

JOHANNES W. ROHEN, M.D.
Full Professor of Anatomy
Head of the Department of Anatomy
University of Erlangen-Nürnberg
Erlangen, West-Germany

Second edition

UNIVERSITY PARK PRESS Baltimore
IGAKU-SHOIN Ltd. Tokyo

Library of Congress Cataloging in Publication Data

Yokochi, Chihiro, 1918 —
    Photographic anatomy of the human body.

    1. Anatomy, Human—Atlases. I. Rohen, Johannes
Wilhelm. II. Title. [DNLM; 1. Anatomy—Atlases.
QS17 Y54j]
QM25.Y613 1977   611'.0022'2   77-4976
ISBN 0-8391-1104-5

PUBLISHERS
© Second edition 1978 and First edition 1969 by IGAKU-SHOIN Ltd., 5-24-3 Hongo, Bunkyo-ku, Tokyo.
    Sole distribution rights for the United States, Canada and Europe including the United Kingdom granted to
    UNIVERSITY PARK PRESS, 233 East Redwood Street, Baltimore, Maryland 21202

Printed in Japan

Preface to the second edition

The Japanese edition of Professor Yokochi's monochrome photographic atlas of human anatomy was first published in 1962. The original volume, revised and enlarged with color photographs, appeared in its first English edition in 1969. Both volumes were favorably received and have achieved international recognition.

In light of the success of the two earlier editions and in response to the expanding interest and need for knowledge of the anatomical structure of human organs and organ systems on the part of medical specialists, physicians, paramedical professionals, and laymen, this second English edition of the atlas has now been completed. As was true of the earlier English edition, the figures in this new atlas are photographs, predominantly in color, which vividly illustrate the finer structures of organ tissues as well as the interrelationship among organs. The excellence of these photographic representations in comparison with the drawings characteristic of more conventional anatomical textbooks can hardly be exaggerated.

In this second English edition the nomenclature has been increased. New color photographs of anatomical preparations have been included, especially in the chapters on the skeletal, muscular, circulatory and nervous systems. This edition is further distinguished by the addition in selected chapters of a schematic outline of the organ system, based on the work of Professor Rohen and taken from his *Textbook of Functional Anatomy*. The richness and clarity characteristic of the original atlases have been enhanced by this supplemental material.

The authors are grateful to those who have so generously supported their efforts in the preparation of this second English edition. It is hoped that this expanded and refined atlas will stimulate the reader's interest and augment his/her knowledge of human anatomy.

January 1978   The Authors

Preface to the first edition

Some fifteen years ago, the author compiled the Japanese edition of this photographic atlas of anatomy. It has been in pressing demand ever since its publication and is perhaps the only work approachable for those in the paramedical fields, such as nurses, x-ray technicians, and hygienic specialists. This does not by any means imply that the content of this work is more rudimentary than the college textbooks designed for medical students. On the contrary, it contains a wealth of items of interest to medical specialists and physicians. Furthermore, it is useful to the general readers as well, as it illustrates the mysteries of the human body in an exceptionally vivid and life-like manner.

Ever since its first publication in 1962, the Japanese edition of this atlas has been accorded a favorable reception. In this new English edition, many of the monochrome pictures have been replaced by color photographs and parts of the text have been considerably revised. This atlas enables us to appreciate the general structure of the human body through vivid specimens enormously different from those valid illustrations seen in conventional textbooks.

A special cordiality of Dr. K. Takahashi, Associate Professor, who has kindly supplied his invaluable specimen of the fetus for this atlas is gratefully acknowledged.

The contribution of Mr. O. Tobiume who has prepared the specimens of general muscles of the human body in this atlas cannot be exaggerated.

Tokyo, October 1969   CHIHIRO YOKOCHI

Contents

BONES

Structure of Bones

The exterior surface of a bone is hard and solid, while the interior is hollow to conserve weight. The space within is filled with marrow. Marrow in an infant or youngster's bone is red ("red marrow") due to the red blood corpuscles abundantly produced within. The corpuscles thus produced are ejected through the nutrient foramen. With advancing age, the red marrow is gradually replaced by fat due to the lowering of hematopoiesis, turning the marrow into yellow ("yellow marrow").

The epiphyses of long bones such as the femur are not hollow but reinforced by the spongy bone, which is also filled with marrow. The interior of short bones such as the vertebra is completely occupied by the spongy bone, leaving no hollow space (cf. p. 6). Even in adulthood these do not turn yellow, since hematopoiesis continues.

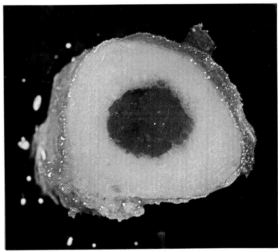

Red marrow

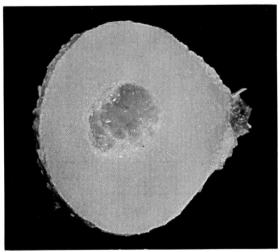

Yellow marrow

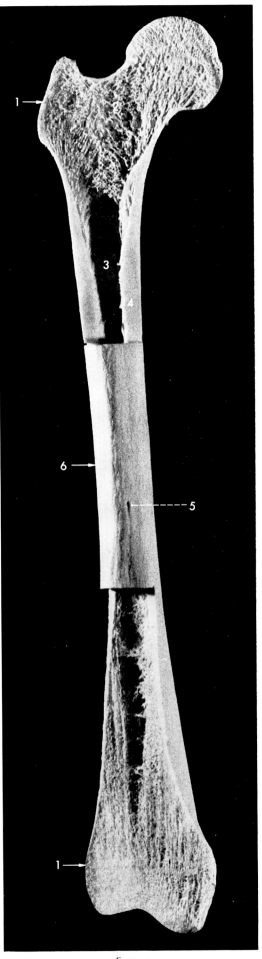

Femur

1. epiphysis	**2.** spongy bone
3. medullary cavity	**4.** compact bone
5. nutrient foramen	**6.** diaphysis

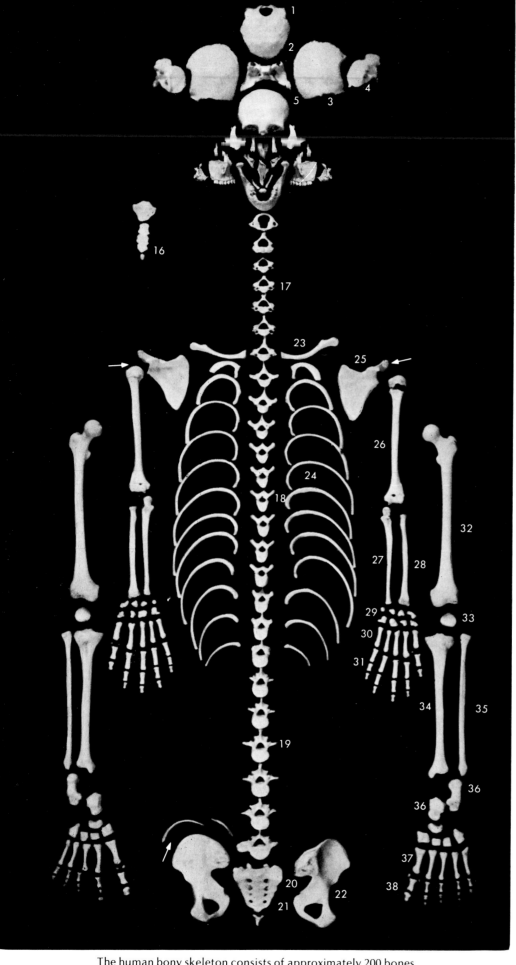

The human bony skeleton consists of approximately 200 bones.

The Bony Skeleton of the Entire Human Body Disassembled

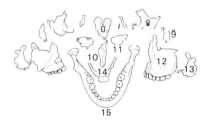

The items composing the human skeleton are as follows;

Vertebrae:	free	24	
	sacral	5	31 — 37
	coccygeal	2 — 6	
Skull		23	
Axial (exclusive of the upper two)		25	
Upper limbs		64	
Lower limbs		62	
Total			205 — 211

The above figures are flexible, since, for instance, the number of coccyx varies according to the individual. Furthermore, opinions vary as to whether the auditory ossicles should be counted. Moreover, as age advances, there are many cases in which the border of the bones is agglutinated.

1. Occipital bone
2. Sphenoid bone
3. Parietal bone
4. Temporal bone
5. Frontal bone
6. Ethmoid bone
7. Nasal bone
8. Zygomatic bone
9. Lacrimal bone
10. Vomer
11. Inferior concha
12. Maxillary bone
13. Palatine bone
14. Hyoid bone
15. Mandible
16. Sternum
17. Cervical vertebrae
18. Thoracic vertebrae
19. Lumbar vertebrae
20. Sacrum
21. Coccyx
22. Hip bone
23. Clavicle
24. Ribs
25. Scapula
26. Humerus
27. Ulna
28. Radius
29. Carpal bones
30. Metacarpals
31. Phalanges
32. Femur
33. Patella
34. Tibia
35. Fibula
36. Tarsus
37. Metatarsals
38. Phalanges
Arrows: Epiphyses

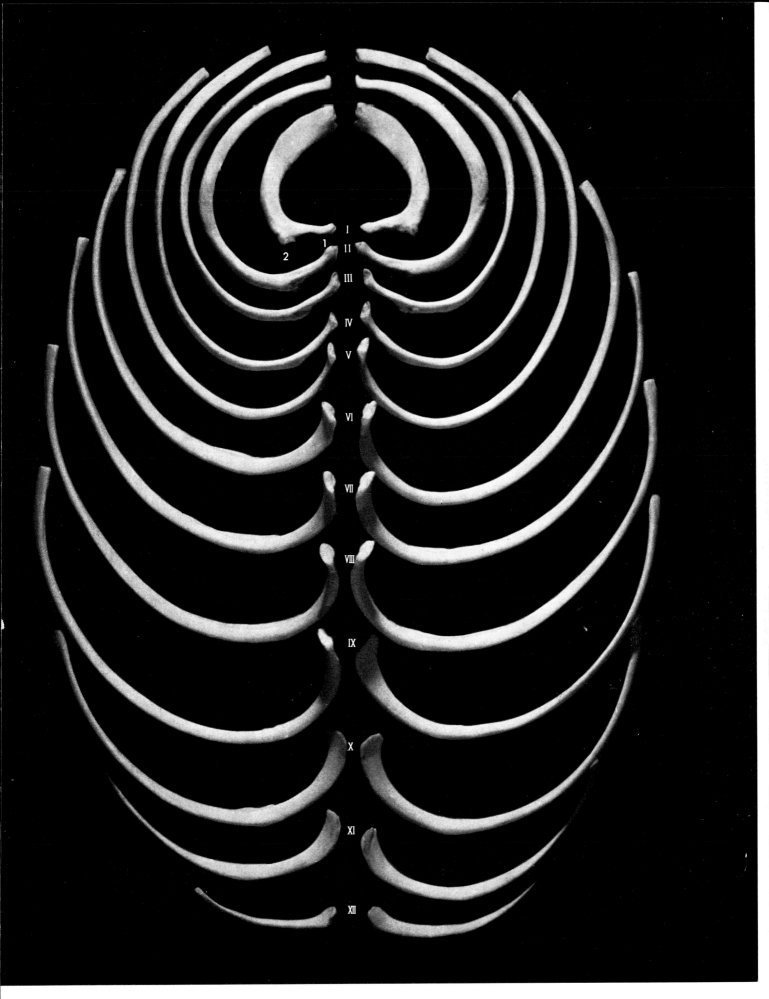

I
II
III
IV
V
VI
VII
VIII
IX
X
XI
XII

1
2

RIBS

1. Head   **2.** Tubercle
The head and tubercle articulated with vertebra.

COMPLETE VIEW OF SKELETON

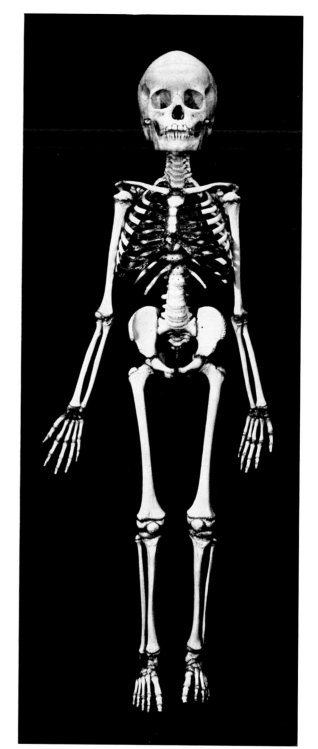

Child's skeleton

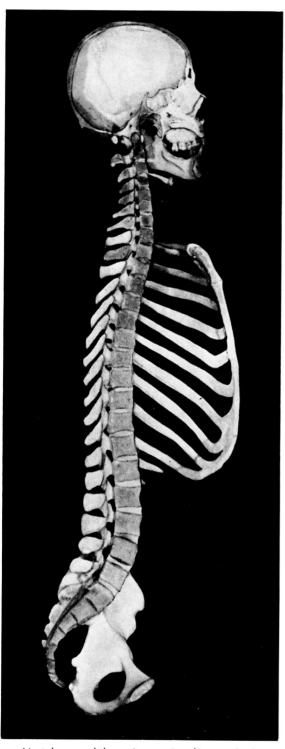

Vertebrae and thoracic cage (median section)

The thorax contains a thoracic cavity, which is filled with the lung and heart, and its lower margin is bounded by a diaphragm. Each rib joins the sternum by a bridge of the costal cartilage. Eleventh and twelfth ribs are very short in length and their ventral ends are free.

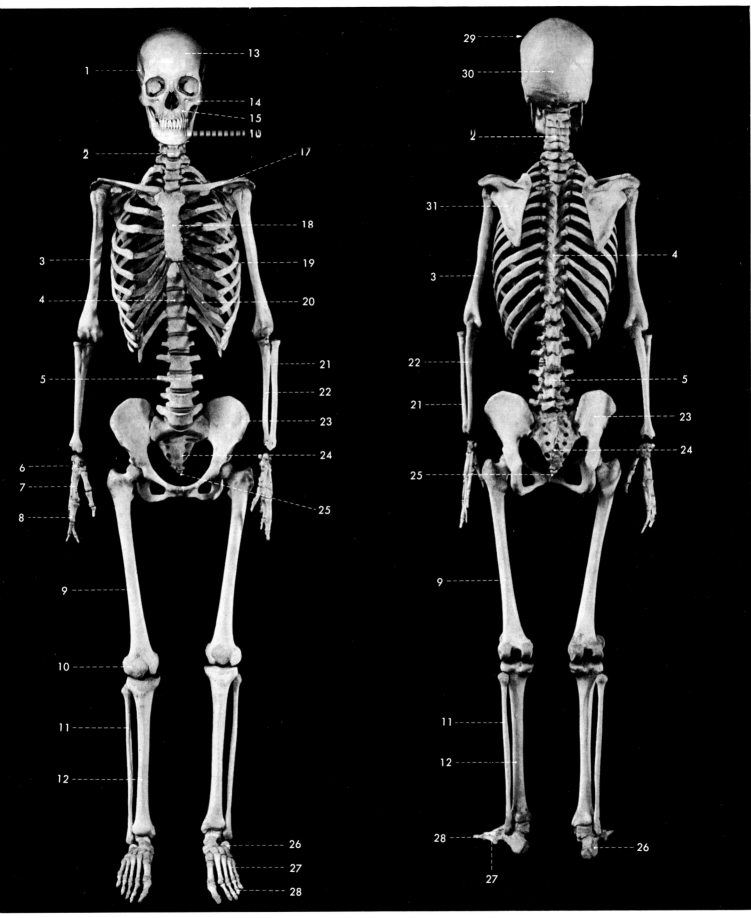

Ventral view   Dorsal view (Female)

1. temporal bone   2. cervical vertebrae   3. humerus   4. thoracic vertebrae   5. lumbar vertebrae   6. carpals
7. metacarpals   8. phalanges   9. femur   10. patella   11. fibula   12. tibia   13. frontal b.   14. zygomatic b.
15. maxilla   16. mandible   17. clavicle   18. sternum   19. ribs   20. costal cartilage   21. radius   22. ulna
23. hip b.   24. sacrum   25. coccyx   26. tarsals   27. metatarsals   28. phalanges   29. parietal b.   30. occipital b.
31. scapula

VERTEBRAE

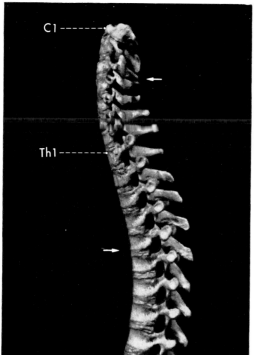

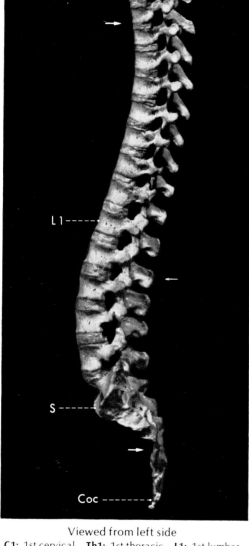

Cervical
curvature

Thoracic
curvature

Lumbar
curvature

Sacro-
coccygeal
curvature

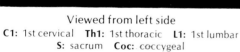
Viewed from left side
C1: 1st cervical **Th1:** 1st thoracic **L1:** 1st lumbar
S: sacrum **Coc:** coccygeal

The vertebral curvature in the embryo presents a simple curve due to the ventriflex posture in the uterus. However, when the infant after birth reaches the stage of assuming the upright position, the vertebral column forms a sigmoid curve as shown above. This curvature helps to prevent direct impact upon the brain in case of a fall, since it functions as a buffer to protect the head.

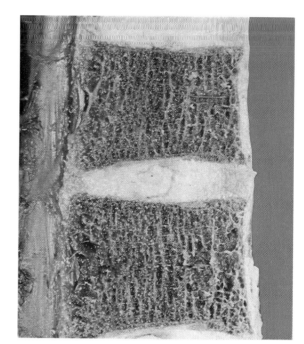

Median section of the vertebral column

Anterior view (lumbar and sacrum)

The intervertebral discs, which are flat elastic cartilages interposed between the vertebrae, permit the vertebral column to be bent or twisted to some extent. Each of the vertebrae is also interconnected by strong ligaments.

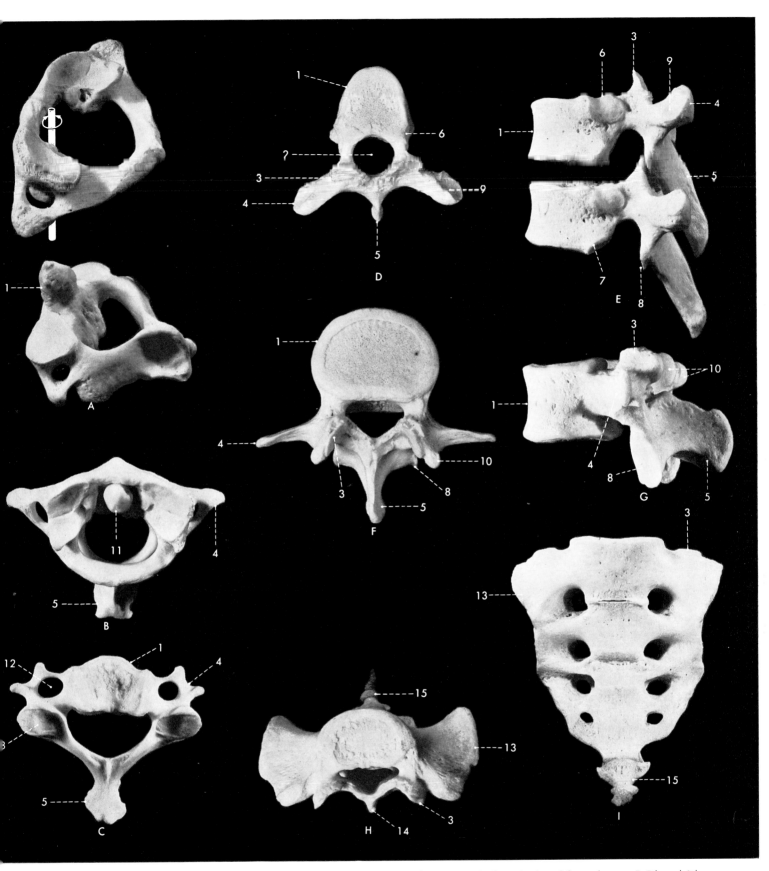

A: Atlanto-axial articulation   **B:** Viewed from above   **C:** 4th cervical from above   **D:** 7th thoracic viewed from above   **E:** 7th and 8th thoracic viewed from left side   **F:** 3rd lumbar viewed from above   **G:** 3rd lumbar viewed from left side   **H:** Sacrum and coccyx viewed from above   **I:** Sacrum and coccyx viewed from front

1. body **2.** vertebral foramen **3.** superior articular process **4.** transverse process **5.** spinous process **6.** sup. costal facet **7.** inf. costal facet **8.** inf. articular process **9.** facet for costal tubercle **10.** mammilary process **11.** dens **12.** transverse foramen **13.** ala **14.** median sacral crest **15.** coccyx

The 2nd cervical vertebra has a dens projecting upward, which is inserted into the 1st cervical vertebra, serving as a pivot for rotation. The 1st cervical vertebra supports the skull. It derives its name "Atlas" from a god of that name in Greek mythology, who is supposed to have supported the earth. The sacral vertebra is a bone formed by agglutination of 5 separate bones. Further, the transverse process of the cervical vertebrae are formed by fusion of the transverse processes in proper and the ribs. The vertebral artery runs through the foramen in the transverse processes.

SKULL

The skull consists of 23 bones of 15 different kinds.

The cranium containing the brain comprises the following bones:

Occipital bone	1	Ethmoid bone	1
Sphenoid bone	1	Inferior nasal concha	2
Temporal bone	2	Lacrimal bone	2
Parietal bone	2	Nasal bone	2
Frontal bone	1	Vomer	1

The bones of the face are:

Maxilla	2	Mandible	1
Palatine bone	2	Hyoid bone	1
Zygomatic bone	2		

The skull is generally disassembled by steeping it in water after filling it with beans. The pressure of the swelling beans loosens the sutures. This method, however, can be employed only for skulls of infants up to the age of approximately 15. Adult sutures are difficult to separate, not to mention those of aged persons, which almost disappear due to synostosis (see p. 10).

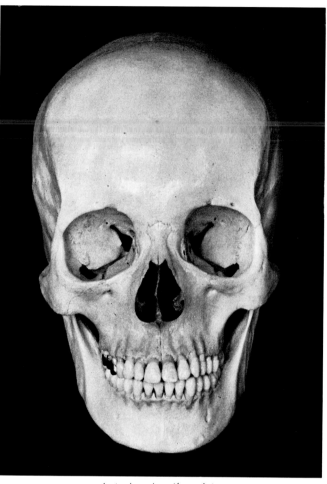

Anterior view (female)

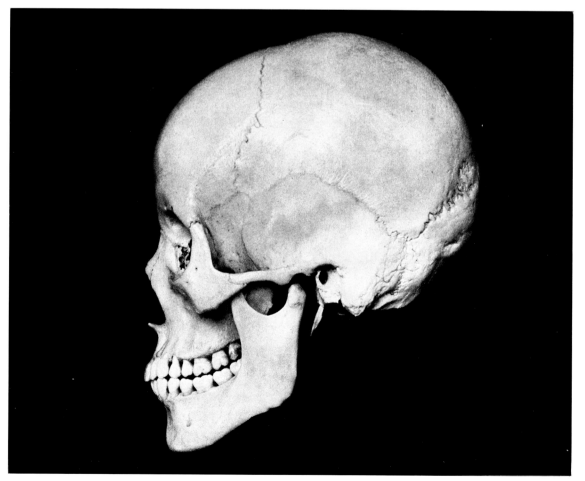

Lateral view

Skull Disassembled (lateral view)

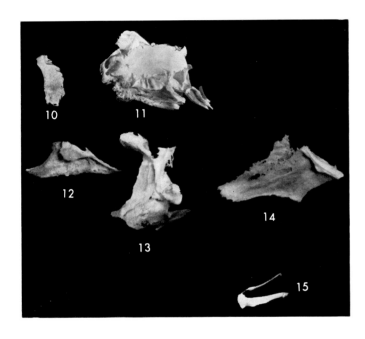

1. frontal bone
2. sphenoid bone
3. zygomatic bone
4. nasal bone
5. maxilla
6. temporal bone
7. occipital bone
8. parietal bone
9. mandible
10. lacrimal bone
11. ethmoid bone
12. inferior nasal concha
13. palatine bone
14. vomer
15. hyoid bone

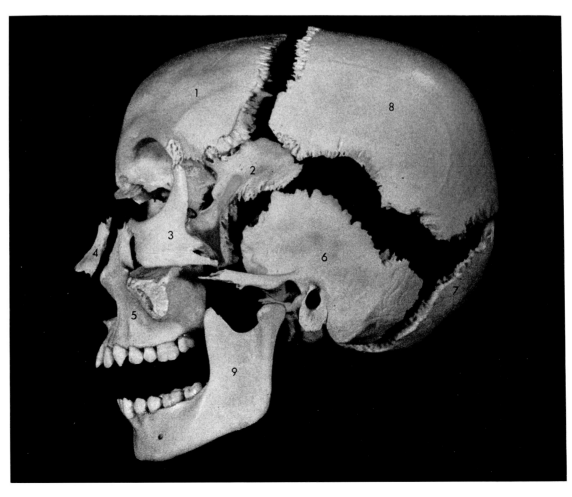

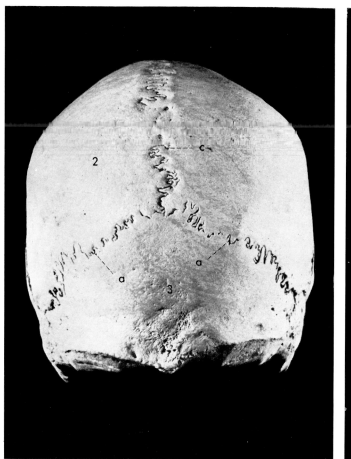

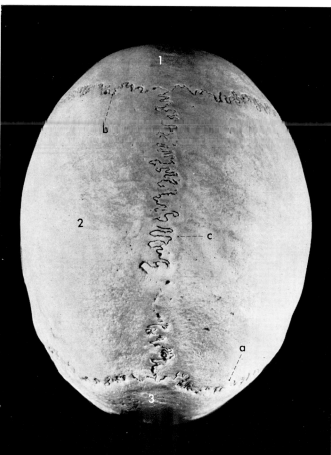

Posterior view   Superior view

1. frontal bone **2.** parietal bone **3.** occipital bone **a.** lambdoid suture **b.** coronal suture **c.** sagittal suture

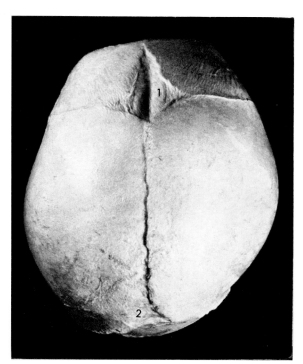

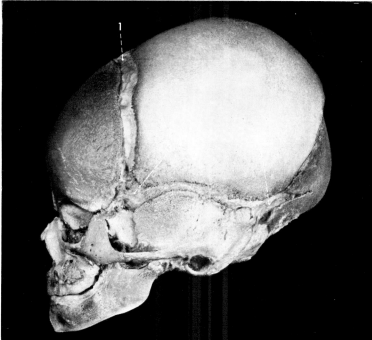

Skull of infant at birth

1. frontal fontanelle **2.** occipital fontanelle **3.** sphenoid (antero-lateral) fontanelle **4.** mastoid (postero-lateral) fontanelle

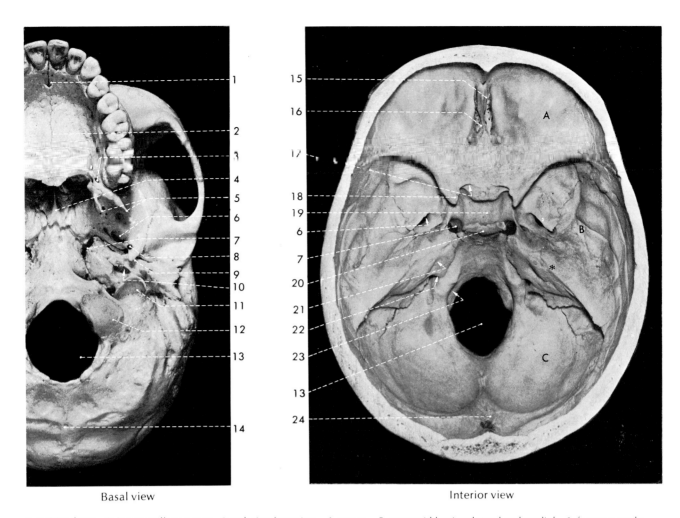

Basal view   Interior view

1. incisive fossa 2. intermaxillary suture 3. palatine foramina 4. vomer 5. pterygoid lamina; lateral and medial 6. foramen-ovale
7. foramen lacerum 8. foramen spinosum 9. styloid process 10. external carotid foramen 11. jugular fossa 12. occipital condyle
13. foramen magnum 14. external occipital protuberance 15. crista galli 16. cribriform plate of ethmoid 17. optic canal 18. anterior
clinoid process 19. hypophysial fossa 20. post. clinoid process 21. int. acoustic meatus 22. jugular foramen 23. hypoglossal canal
24. confluens of sinuses

A. anterior fossa B. middle fossa C. posterior fossa * arcuate eminence

The skull is composed of numerous flat bones tightly interlocked like an elaborately-constructed wooden box. This type of joint is called serrate suture (cf. p. 16).

At the stages of fetus and infant, the bones of the cranial vault are joined by connective tissues, which allow modification of the skull to facilitate its passage through the birth canal. There are also several unossified areas covered by membrane, the most representative of which are the anterior and posterior fontanelles. Whereas the former does not close until 2 or 3 years after birth, the latter shuts within 6 to 12 months after birth. The former is important for obstetricians, since, by feeling it, they can determine the direction in which the infant is facing in the womb. At this stage the frontal bone is still divided into two.

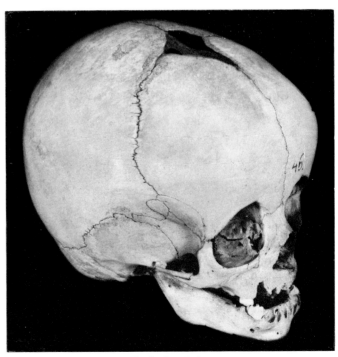

Skull of an infant

PELVIS

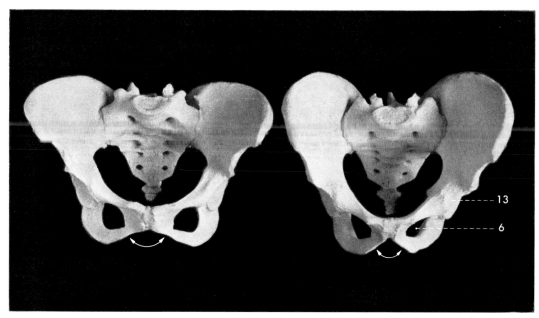

female   Anterior view   male

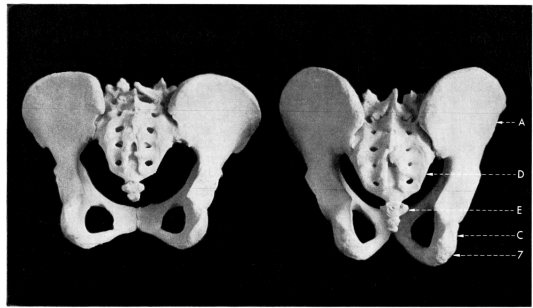

female   Posterior view   male

A. ilium
B. pubis
C. ischium
D. sacrum
E. coccyx

1. iliac crest
2. ant. sup. iliac spine
3. ant. inf. iliac spine
4. acetabulum
5. pubic tubercle
6. obturator foramen
7. ischial tuberosity
8. lesser sciatic notch
9. spine of ischium
10. greater sciatic notch
11. post. inf. iliac spine
12. post. sup. iliac spine
13. iliopubic eminence
14. iliac fossa
15. pelvic cavity
16. pecten
17. symphysis
18. arcuate line

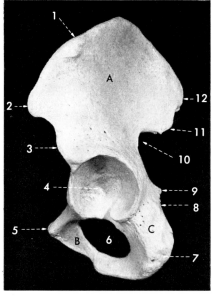

Hip bone, lateral view (left)

Differences according to Sex

The most conspicuous difference between the skeletons of the two sexes is found in the pelvis as shown above, the female pelvis is broader and lower in height than that of the male. Furthermore, the pelvic cavity of the male is heart-shaped, whereas that of the female is much broader and transversely oval.

Moreover the subpubic angle of the female pelvis presents a gentle arch-like curve, while that of a male forms a sharp angle. The female pelvis is thus built to facilitate the passage of the fetus through the maternal channel.

The pelvis consists of the left and right coxae (hip bones) and a sacrum. The coxae are formed through fusion of the ilium, ischium, and pubis. At the converging point of the three bones, there is the acetabulum, into which the head of the femur is inserted.

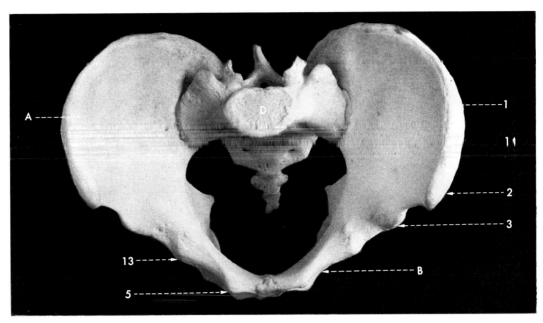

Superior view (male)

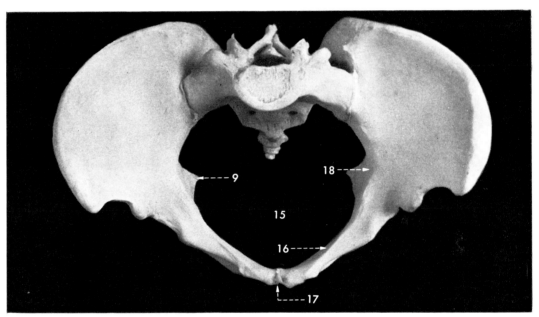

Superior view (female)

The Measurement of the Dimension and Capacity of Pelvis (pelvimetry)

The pelvimetry for the female pelvis is important for anthropology as well as for obstetrics. The measurement is usually made outside the body in the living human and sometimes made using the X-ray photograph.

Various diameters of female pelvis
a. anteroposterior diameter (true conjugate)
b. obstetrical conjugate
c. diagonal conjugate
d. transverse diameter
e. arcuate line

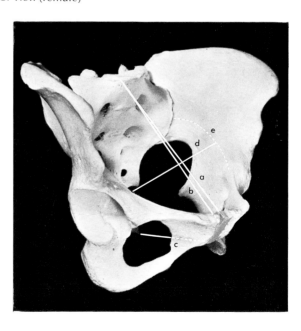

BONES OF THE EXTREMITIES

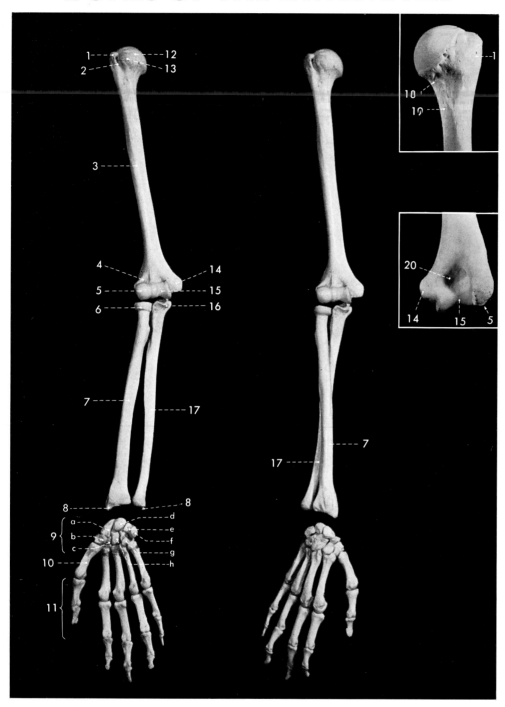

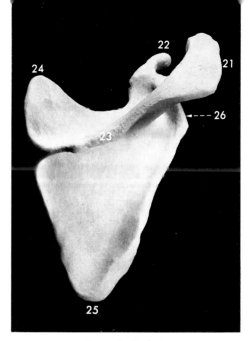

Scapula (right)
(dorsal surface)

Supination (palmar view)   Pronation (dorsal view)

Upper extremity (right)

The natural position of the hands and wrists is midway between supination and pronation. In full supination the radius and ulna are parallel, while in full pronation, they are crossed. In this way, although the wrist joint is not rotative against the forearm, it rotates against the axis of the humerus. (Insets: dorsal view)

1. greater tubercle   **2.** intertubercular sulcus   **3.** groove for radial nerve   **4.** lateral epicondyle   **5.** capitulum   **6.** head   **7.** radius   **8.** styloid process   **9-a.** scaphoid **b.** trapezium   **c.** trapezoideum   **d.** lunate   **e.** triquetral   **f.** pisiform   **g.** hamte **h.** capitate   **10.** metacarpus   **11.** phalanges   **12.** head   **13.** lesser tubercle   **14.** medial epicondyle   **15.** trochlea   **16.** coronoid process   **17.** ulna   **18.** anatomical neck **19.** surgical neck   **20.** olecranon fossa   **21.** acromion   **22.** coracoid process   **23.** spine **24.** sup. angle   **25.** inf. angle   **26.** glenoid cavity   **27.** head   **28.** neck   **29.** lesser trochanter   **30.** medial epicondyle   **31.** med. condyle   **32.** tibia   **33.** med. malleolus **34-a.** calcaneus   **b.** talus   **c.** navicular   **d.** cuneiform   **e.** cuboid   **35.** greater trochanter **36.** femur   **37.** lateral epicondyle   **38.** patella   **39.** head   **40.** fibula   **41.** lat. malleolus   **42.** metatarsus   **43.** phalanges   **44.** med. condyle   **45.** intercondyloid fossa **46.** lat. condyle

14

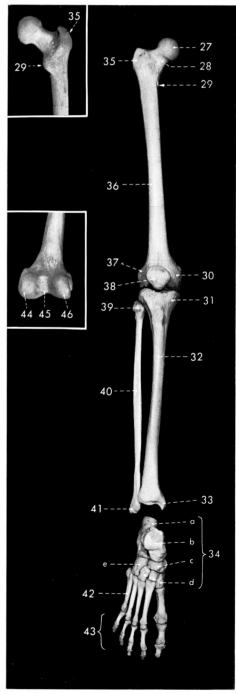

Lower extremity (right)

JOINTS

In the case of a movable joint, the head of one bone presents a convex articular surface, while that of the other a concave glenoid cavity. Their surfaces are covered by a layer of glassy hyaline cartilage. The opposed ends of the bones are connected by a sheath-shaped articular capsule composed of connective tissues, which in turn form the joint cavity.

Lining the interior of the joint capsule is the synovial membrane, which secretes the mucous synovial fluid to lubricate the joint. Some joints have intra-articular discs or ligaments (cf. right upper photograph and p.17 "*")

A. femur   **B.** tibia   **C.** fibula
1. lat. collateral lig.   **2.** lat. meniscus   **3.** med. collateral lig.   **4.** ant. cruciate lig.   **5.** med. meniscus   **6.** articular cartilage

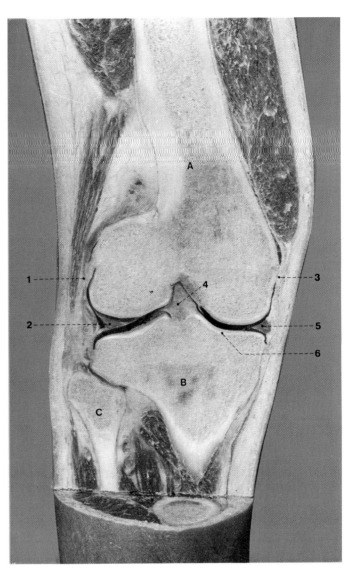

Knee joint (frontal section)

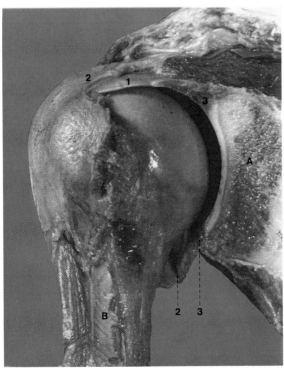

Shoulder joint (muscles are removed.)

A. scapula   **B.** humerus
1. tendon of long head of biceps brachii
2. articular capsule   **3.** glenoidal labrum

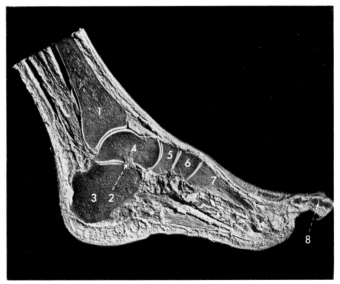

Longitudinal section through the foot, showing the arch of the foot.

1. tibia   **2.** talocalcaneal interosseus lig.   **3.** calcaneus   **4.** talus
5. navicular   **6.** medial cuneiform   **7.** metatarsal   **8.** phalanges

15

Principal Joints
Immovable articulations

1. Fibrous joints
A. Sutures
a. Serrated or dentated suture

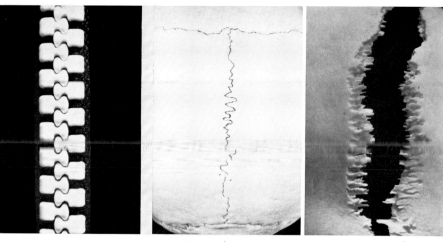

Sagittal suture   separated

b. Squamous or scally suture

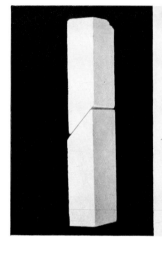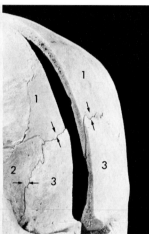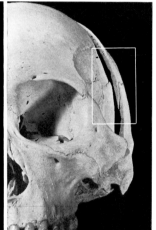

1. parietal bone   2. sphenoid b.   3. squama of temporal b.

c. Harmonia

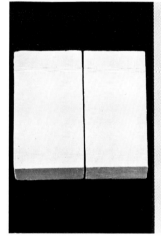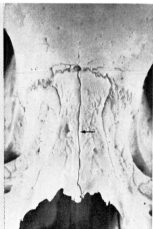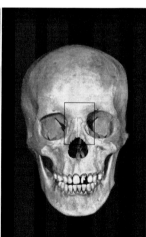

Nasal bones

B. Peg suture

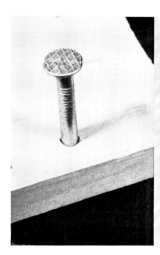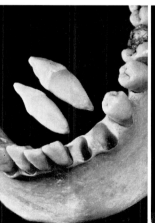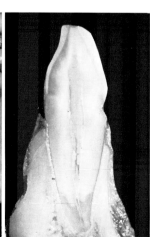

Teeth and alveolar

2. Cartilaginous joints

a. Symphysis (fibrocartilage)

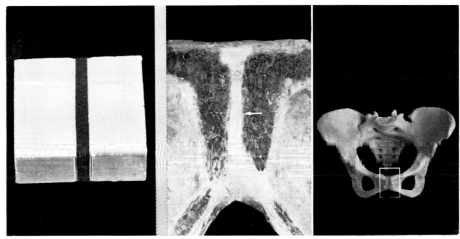

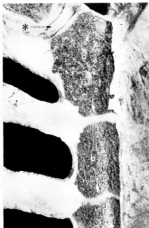
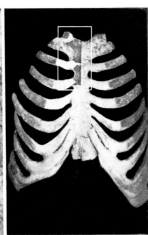

Pubic symphysis

b. Synchondrosis (hyaline cartilage)

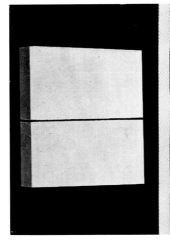
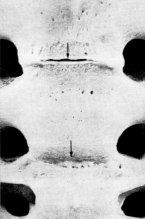
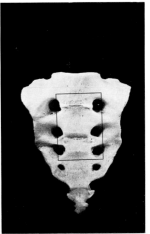

Sternum   **a.** manubrium   **b.** body

3. Osseous joints

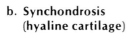

Transverse ridge   Sacrum

---

* articular disc (sternoclavicular joint, *cf.* p. 15)

Synovial joints, articulations (movable joints)

1. Condyloid joint

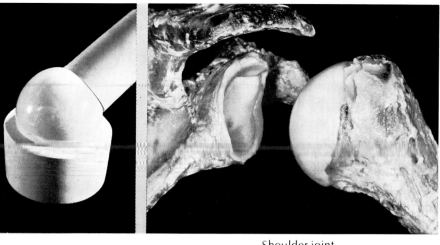

Shoulder joint

2. Ball and socket joint

Hip joint   *glenoid labrum

3. Ellipsoid joint

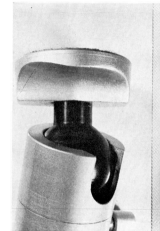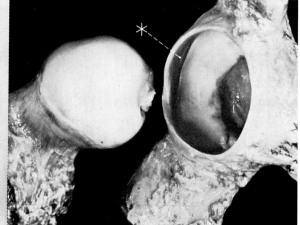

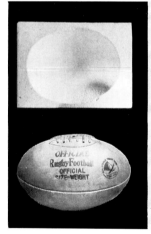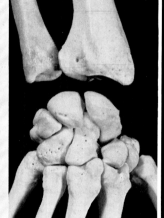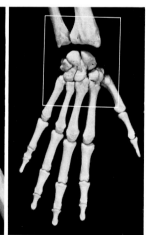

Wrist joint

4. Hinge joint

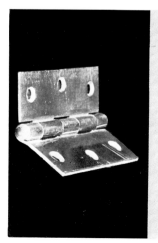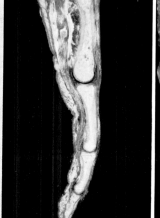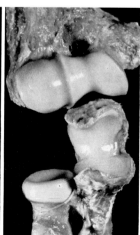

Interphalangeal joint   Elbow joint

5. Pivot joint

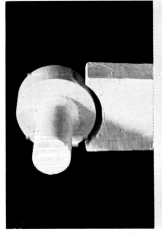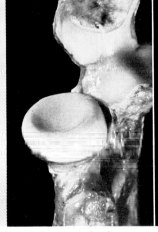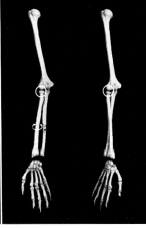

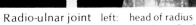

Radio-ulnar joint   left: head of radius
                               right: radial notch of ulna   Supinated   Pronated

6. Cochlear joint

This is a sort of hinge joint, however the difference is that the direction of sulcus at the head of a bone is not vertical to the axis of cylinder; that is to say, it correspond with the screw.

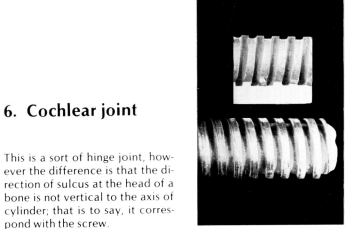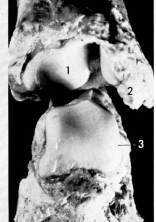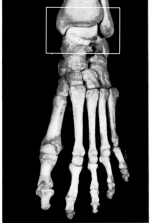

Ankle joint   **1.** tibia   **2.** fibula   **3.** talus

7. Saddle joint

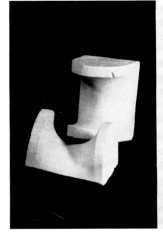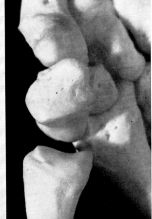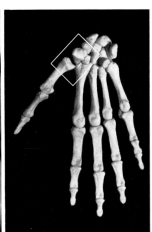

Carpo-metacarpal joint of the thumb

8. Plane joint

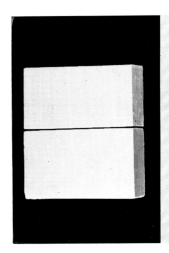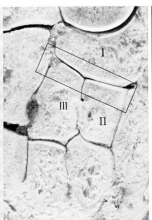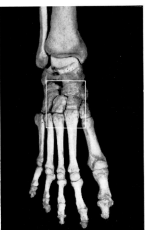

I. navicular, II. intermediate and III. lateral cuneiform

SKELETAL MUSCLES

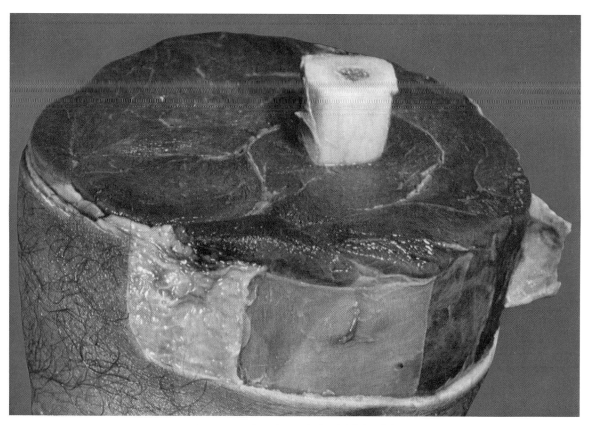

A cross-section through the thigh (male)

1. skin **2.** subcutaneous fat **3.** fascia lata **4.** perimysium
5. muscle **6.** os **7.** periosteum **8.** sciatic nerve **9.** femoral artery
and vein **10.** long saphenous vein
a. rectus femoris **b.** vastus lateralis **c.** vastus medialis **d.** vastus
intermedius **e.** sartorius **f.** biceps femoris **g.** semitendinosus
h. semimembranosus **i.** adductor magnus **j.** adductor longus
k. gracilis

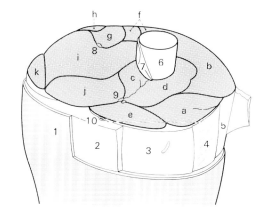

Classification by Muscle Forms

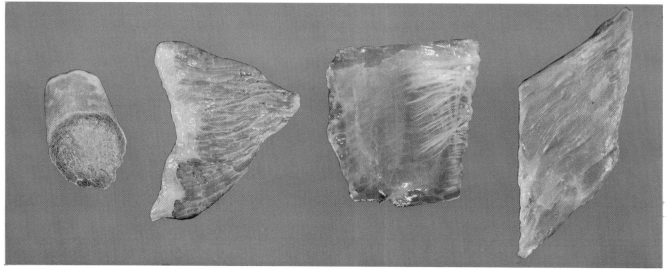

Cylindrical
(teres major)

Triangular
(deltoideus)

Quadrilateral
(pronator quadratus)

Rhomboid
(rhomboideus major)

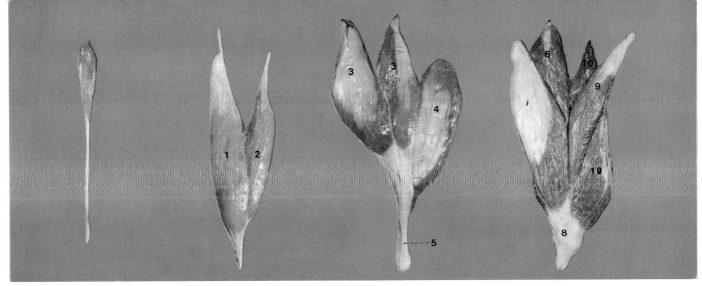

Fusiform
(palmaris longus)

Biceps
(biceps femoris)

Triceps
(triceps surae)

Quadriceps
(quadriceps femoris)

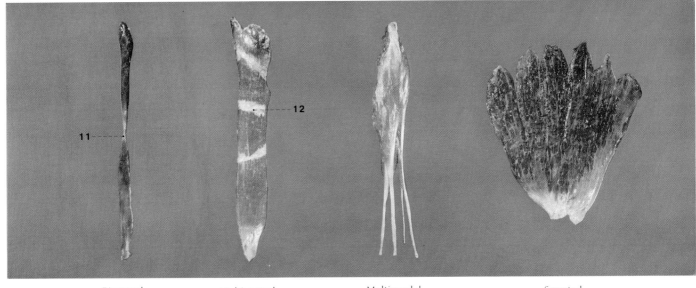

Biventral
(omnohyoid m.)

Multiventral
(rectus abdominis)

Multicaudal
(flexor digitorum prof.)

Serrated
(serratus anterior)

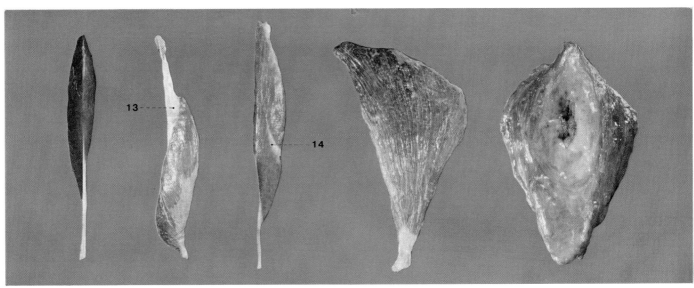

Bipenniform
(tibialis anterior)

Unipenniform
(semimembranosus)

Semitendinous
(semitendinosus)

Broad, flatt m.
(latissimus dorsi)

Ringform
(sphincter ani externus)

1. long head   **2.** short head   **3.** gastrocnemius (medial head, lateral head)   **4.** soleus   **5.** tendon of Achilles   **6.** vastus intermedius   **7.** vastus medialis   **8.** patella   **9.** rectus femoris   **10.** vastus lateralis   **11.** intermediate tendon   **12.** tendinous intersection
13. aponeurosis   **14.** tendinous intersection

Superficial Muscles

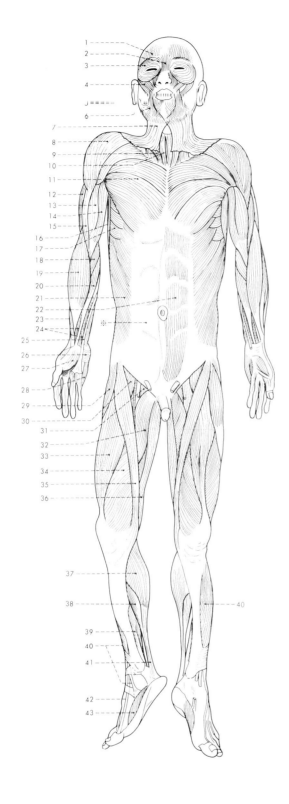

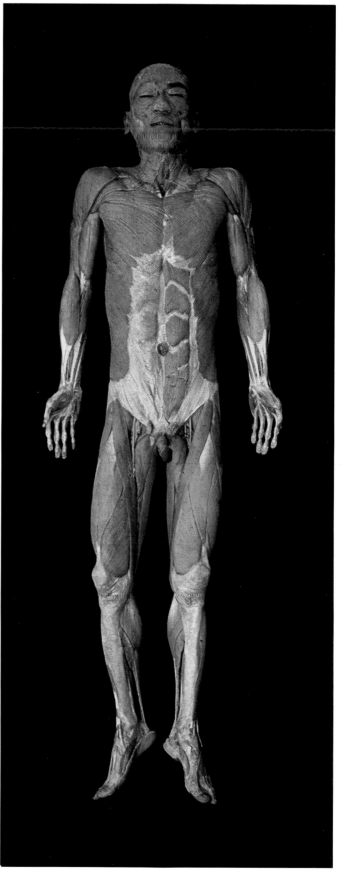

Anterior aspect

1. frontal belly of occipito-frontalis   2. procerus   3. orbicularis oculi   4. zygomaticus major, minor, levator anguli oris, levator labii superioris alaeque nasi   5. depressor labii inferioris   6. risorius, depressor anguli oris   7. platysma   8. deltoid   9. sternocleidomastoid   10. sterno-hyoid 11. pectoralis major   12. lateral head of triceps   13. long head of biceps   14. short head of biceps   15. brachialis   16. latissimus dorsi   17. serratus anterior   18. pronator teres   19. brachioradialis   20. flexor carpi radialis   21. external abdominal oblique m.   22. rectus abdominis   23. abductor pollicis longus   24. flexor digitorum superficialis   25. palmaris longus   26. palmaris brevis   27. thenar eminence   28. abductor digiti minimi   29. tensor fasciae latae   30. iliopsoas   31. pectineus   32. adductor longus   33. rectus femoris   34. vastus medialis   35. sartorius 36. gracilis   37. gastrocnemius   38. soleus   39. flexor digitorum longus   40. tibialis anterior   41. tendo calcaneus   42. ext. hallucis longus 43. abductor hallucis   * aponeurosis of external oblique (rectus sheath)

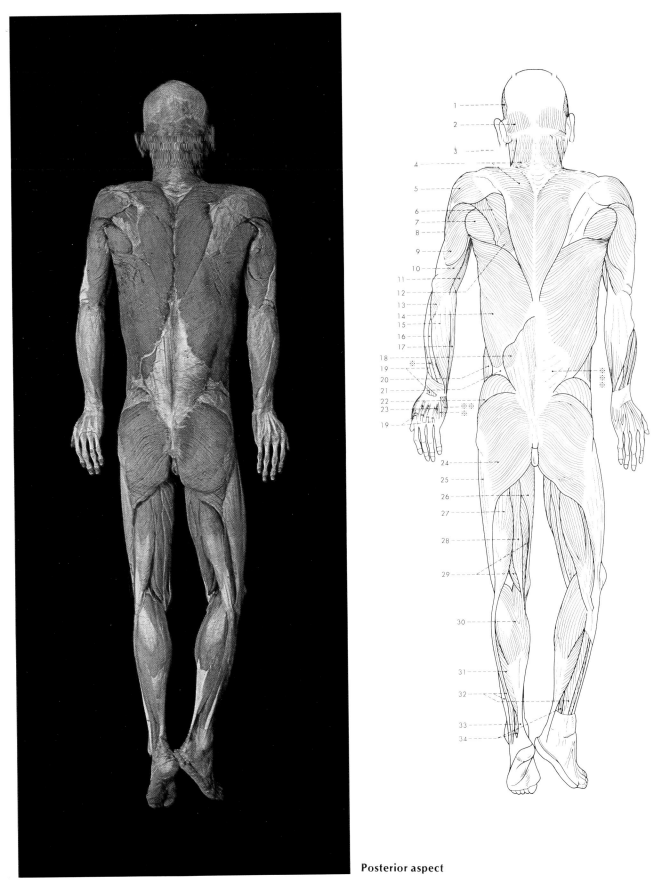

Posterior aspect

1. temporalis m.   2. occipital belly of occipito-frontalis   3. sternocleidomastoideus   4. trapezius   5. deltoid   6. infraspinatus   7. teres major
8. lateral head of triceps   9. long head of triceps   10. medial head of triceps   11. brachialis   12. rhomboideus major   13. anconeus   14. latissimus dorsi   15. flexor carpi ulnaris   16. extensor carpi ulnaris   17. flexor digitorum superficialis   18. serratus posterior inferior   19. extensor digitorum (communis)   20. ext. abdominal oblique   21. lumbar triangle   22. gluteus medius   23. dorsal interosseous   24. gluteus maximus   25. iliotibial tract of fascia lata   26. gracilis   27. biceps femoris (long head)   28. semitendinosus   29. semimembranosus   30. gastrocnemius   31. soleus
32. peroneus longus   33. tendo calcaneus   34. peroneus brevis   * ext. digiti minimi   ** abductor digiti minimi   *** lumbodorsal fascia

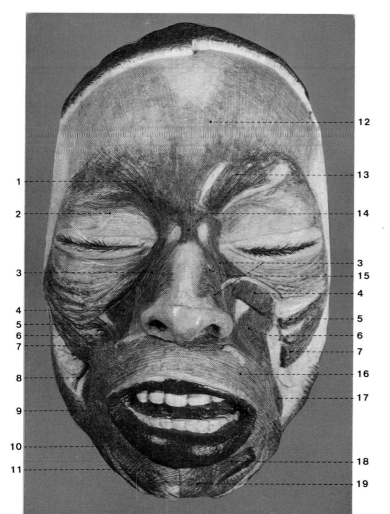

Muscles of Facial Expression

The muscles of facial expression developed from muscles for opening and shutting the facial vents such as the eyes, the nostrils and the mouth. The insertions of these muscles, therefore, converge upon the areas surrounding these vents.

While ordinary muscles originate from and are inserted into bones, the facial muscles are exceptional; they originate from bones but are inserted into the facial skin so as to move the latter. Such muscles are referred to as cutaneous muscles. Their function may be clearly observed, for example, on the neck skin of a horse as it twitches to chase away flies.

1. depressor supercilli
2. orbicularis oculi
3. levator labii superioris alaeque nasi
4. levator labii sup.
5. zygomaticus minor
6. levator anguli oris
7. zygomaticus major
8. risorius
9. platysma
10. depressor anguli oris
11. depressor labii inf.
12. frontal belly of occipito-frontalis
13. corrugator supercilli
14. procerus
15. transverse part of nasalis (compressor naris)
16. orbicularis oris
17. buccinator
18. orbicularis oris (incisivus labii inf.)
19. mentalis

Muscles of Mastication

There are four muscles for mastication, which take part in biting and chewing. The major part of the temporal muscle, the masseter muscle and the medial pterygoid muscle act in closing the jaw; lateral pterygoid muscle acts in depression and protrusion of the mandibula; and the posterior part of the temporal muscle acts in retraction of the jaw.

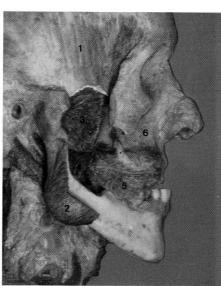

1. temporal
2. masseter
3. lateral pterygoid
4. medial pterygoid
5. buccinator
6. parotid duct

Deep section

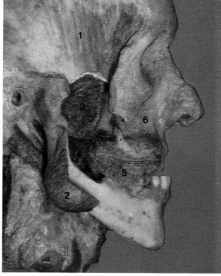

Muscles of upper Extremity (deep layer)

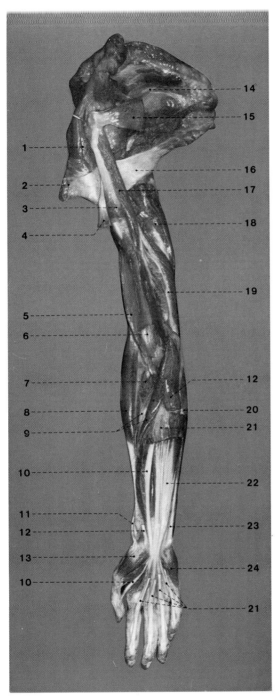

Front of right upper extremity

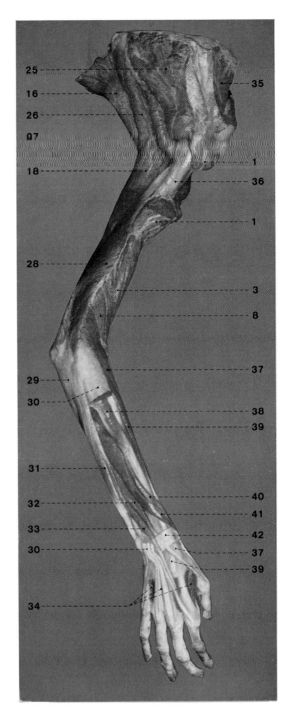

Back of right upper extremity

Muscles that have the origin in the forearm and terminate in the digitus are used in tasks that require strength such as lifting heavy articles, while smaller muscles in the hand are used in finer tasks such as in writing.

1. deltoideus 2. pectoralis major 3. long head (biceps brachii) 4. short head (biceps brachii) 5. brachialis 6. biceps brachii 7. supinator 8. brachioradialis 9. pronator teres 10. flexor pollicis longus 11. abductor pollicis longus 12. flexor carpi radialis 13. muscles of thenar eminence 14. subscapularis 15. pectoralis minor 16. latissimus dorsi 17. coracobrachialis 18. long head (triceps brachii) 19. medial head (triceps brachii) 20. palmaris longus 21. flexor digitorum superficialis 22. flexor digitorum profundus 23. flexor carpi ulnaris 24. muscles of hypothenar eminence 25. infraspinatus 26. teres major 27. teres minor 28. lateral head of triceps brachii 29. anconeus 30. extensor digitorum 31. extensor carpi ulnaris 32. extensor pollicis longus 33. extensor indicis 34. dorsal interossei 35. supraspinatus 36. humerus 37. extensor carpi radialis longus 38. supinator 39. extensor carpi radialis brevis 40. abductor pollicis longus 41. extensor pollicis brevis 42. extensor retinaculum

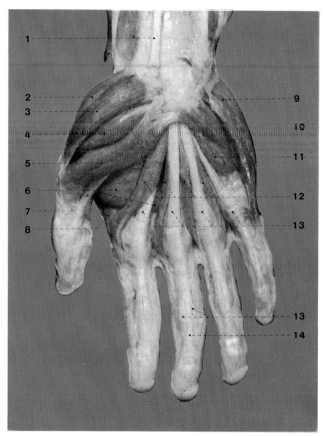

Anterior view of palm of hand. Palmar aponeurosis and palmaris brevis have been removed.

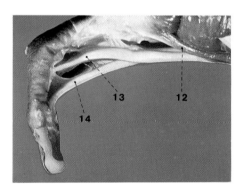

Tendon of flexor digitorum superficialis divides in two and attaches to the middle phalanx. Furthermore, the tendon of flexor digitorum profundus passes through the bifurcation and terminates at the distal phalanx. The finger, therefore, can be bent by the synergistic action of the two. On the other hand, the lumbrical reaches the extensor expansion by passing lateral of the ossa digitorum manus. Its function is to flex the metacarpophalangeal joint while leaving the digitus extended.

1. palmaris longus   2. opponens pollicis   3. abductor pollicis brevis   4. deep head (flexor pollicis brevis)   5. superficial head (flexor pollicis brevis)   6. oblique head and transverse head of abductor pollicis   7. flexor pollicis longus   8. 1st dorsal interosseous   9. abductor digiti minimi   10. flexor digiti minimi   11. opponens digiti minimi   12. lumbrical   13. flexor digitorum superficialis   14. flexor digitorum profundus

Muscles of Lower Extremity (deep layer)

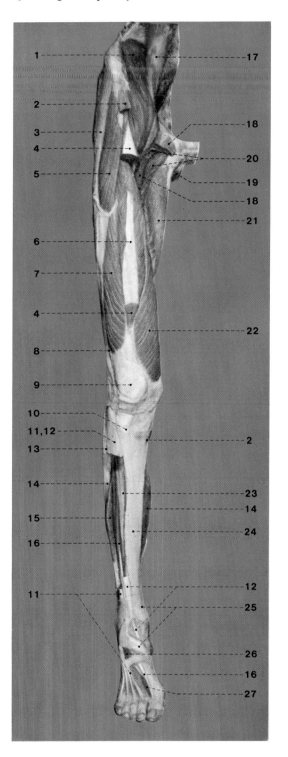

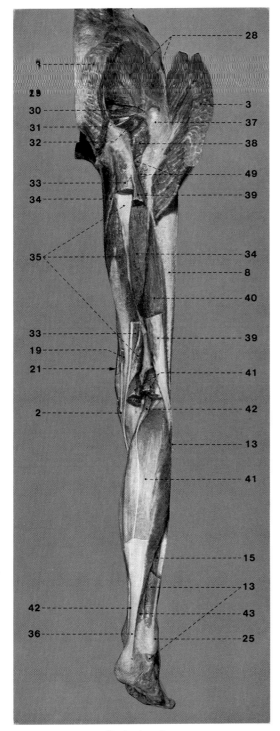

Posterior view

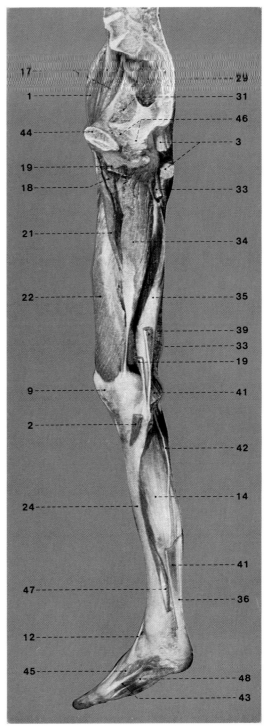

Medial view

1. iliacus 2. sartorius 3. gluteus maximus 4. rectus femoris 5. tensor fasciae latae 6. vastus intermedius 7. vastus lateralis 8. iliotibial band 9. patella 10. tuberosity of the tibia 11. extensor digitorum longus 12. tibialis anterior 13. peroneus longus 14. soleus 15. peroneus brevis 16. extensor hallucis longus 17. psoas major 18. pectineus 19. gracilis 20. obturator externus, adductor brevis 21. adductor longus 22. vastus medialis 23. interosseous membrane 24. tibia 25. sup. and inf. extensor retinaculum 26. ext. hallucis brevis 27. interosseus dorsalis 28. gluteus medius 29. piriformis 30. gemellus superior 31. obturator internus 32. gemellus·inferior 33. semitendinosus 34. adductor magnus 35. semimembranosus 36. tendo calcaneus (Achilles) 37. greater trochanter 38. quadratus femoris 39. biceps femoris (long head) 40. biceps femoris (short head) 41. gastrocnemius 42. plantaris 43. flexor hallucis longus 44. symphysis pubis 45. abductor hallucis 46. levator ani 47. flexor digitorum longus 48. flexor digitorum brevis 49. adductor minimus

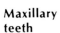

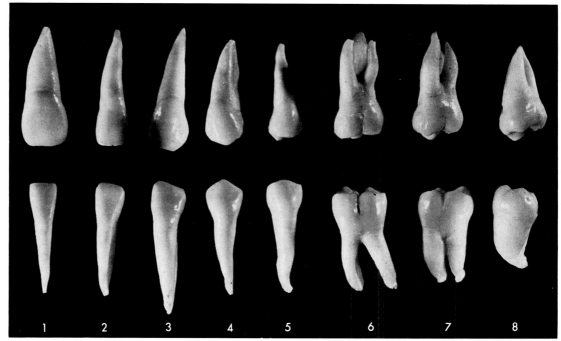

TEETH

Arrangement of the teeth

Dental formula

(8)	7	6	5	4	3	2	1		1	2	3	4	5	6	7	(8)
(8)	7	6	5	4	3	2	1		1	2	3	4	5	6	7	(8)

M_3	M_2	M_1	P_2	P_1	C	I_2	I_1		I_1	I_2	C	P_1	P_2	M_1	M_2	M_3
M_3	M_2	M_1	P_2	P_1	C	I_2	I_1		I_1	I_2	C	P_1	P_2	M_1	M_2	M_3

Among the 8, 5 in front are named successional teeth, because they grow after the deciduation of the milk teeth. The table showing the sort, number and arrangement of the teeth is named a dental formula.

The third molar begins to appear at 19—22 years of age, but some people do not have this kind of teeth. Only in one third of the adults all the third molars are seen.

The permanent arch (outside) and the deciduous arch (inside)

Maxillary teeth

Mandibular teeth

Permanent teeth

1. central incisor (I_1)
2. lateral incisor (I_2)
3. canine
4. first premolar (P_1)
5. second premolar (P_2)
6. first molar (M_1)
7. second molar (M_2)
8. third molar (M_3)

28

Deciduous arch

The milk or deciduous teeth appear from six months to two and a half years after birth, and are replaced by the permanent teeth at six or seven years of age.

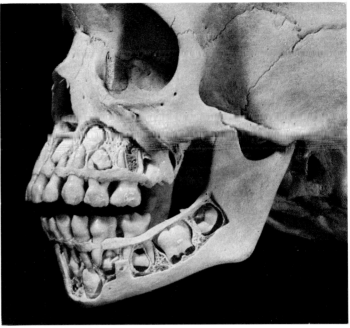

Deciduous and permanent teeth displayed in child's skull
The developing crowns of permanent teeth are embedded under the deciduous teeth.

1. enamel
2. dentin
3. pulp
4. cement
5. root canal
6. crown
7. neck
8. root
9. bone
10. vessels and nerves

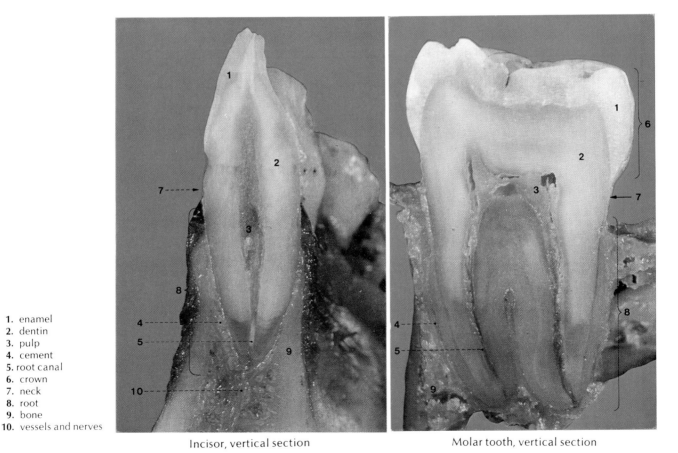

Incisor, vertical section   Molar tooth, vertical section

The root of a tooth is planted in the alveolar bone tissue. Between the bone and the tooth is a periodontium (desmodont) which binds both tissues elastically and even the healthy teeth can be somewhat moved.

Through the canal in the apex of the root, blood vessels and nerve fibers enter the pulp cavity.

TONGUE and PHARYNX

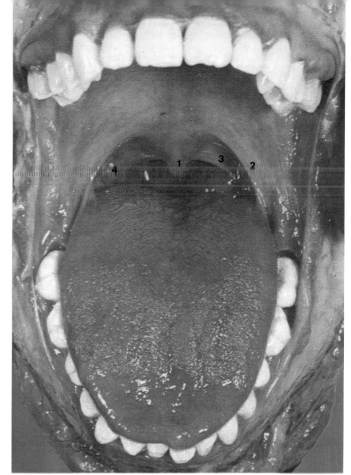

There are three kinds of tonsils: (1) palatine tonsils situated on each side of the fauces (these are what we usually call "tonsils"); (2) a lingual tonsil located at the root of the tongue; and (3) a pharyngeal tonsil situated on the posterior wall of the nasopharynx (this is what is generally called "adenoid") (cf. p. 40)

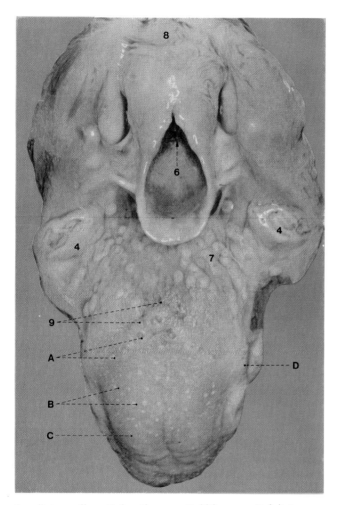

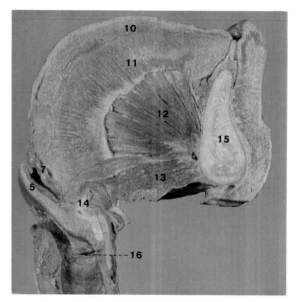

A. vallate papillae   **B.** fungiform p.   **C.** filiform p.   **D.** foliate p.
1. uvula   **2.** palatoglossal arch   **3.** palatopharyngeal arch   **4.** palatine tonsil   **5.** epiglottis   **6.** laryngeal aditus   **7.** lingual follicles (tonsil)   **8.** oesophageal lumen   **9.** foramen caecum and terminal sulcus   **10.** superior longitudinal m.   **11.** vertical and transverse m. **12.** geniglossus m.   **12.** septum   **13.** geniohyoid m.   **14.** hyoid bone   **15.** mandible   **16.** larynx (ventricle)

The front section of the palate is called the hard palate as it contains bone, whereas the rear half is called the soft palate, being composed only of muscles, which have the function of closing the posterior nasal aperture at the time of deglutition.

At the center of the soft palate, there is the uvula, from which two folds named the palatoglossal and palatopharyngeal arches run in the lateral inferior direction on both sides. In between the two arches, there is a palatine tonsil.

The muscles of the tongue

The tongue is an oval-shaped mass of muscles which are instrumental in mastication, deglutition, and phonation, besides controlling the sense of taste. Its surface is covered by a mucous membrane. In the dorsal rear part there is a foramen caecum, which is formed at the embyonic stage by depression of the thyroid gland. With this at the apex, there is a v-shaped sulcus (sulcus terminalis), which divides the tongue into the body in the front and the root in the rear. The end of the tongue is called the tongue-tip. The surface of the tongue is covered with innumerable papillae.

ESOPHAGUS and STOMACH

The muscles of the esophagus consist of striated voluntary muscles (skeletal muscles) in the upper half and smooth involuntary muscles (splanchnic muscles) in the lower half, and a mixture of both types in the intermediary part. The muscular coat comprises circular muscles in the interior and longitudinal muscles in the exterior layers.

Food is not carried down into the stomach by gravity but rather through the peristaltic movement of the esophagus. Man, therefore, can drink water even in the inverted position. The mucous membrane, similar to the oral cavity, consists of strong stratified squamous epithelium, in which there are mucous glands so as to facilitate the slipping of food. The esophagus does not secrete any digestive juice but only mucous. Ordinarily it is depressed ventro-dorsally and closed.

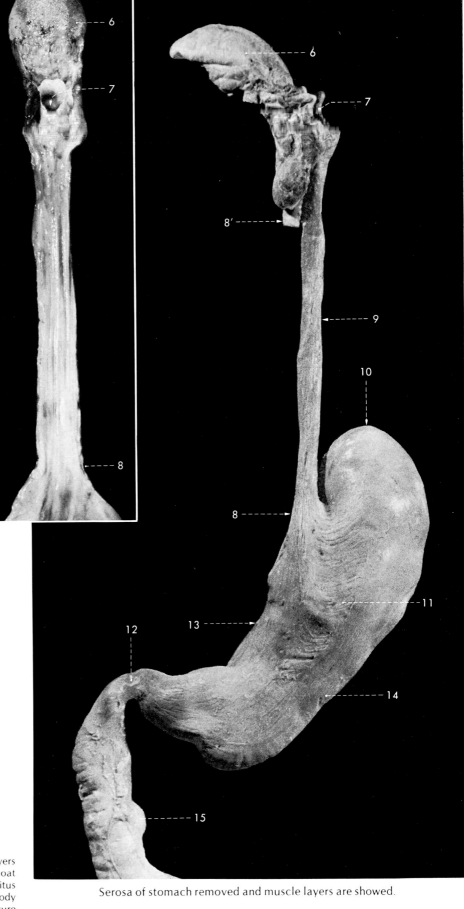

Serosa of stomach removed and muscle layers are showed.

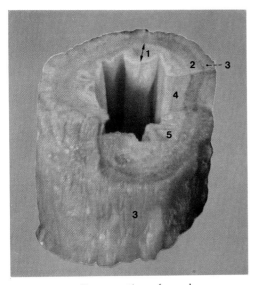

Cross-section of esophagus
Adventitious coat is removed.

1. mucous membrane 2. inner circular muscle layers
3. outer longitudinal muscle layers 4. submucous coat
5. esophageal glands 6. tongue 7. laryngeal aditus
8. cardia 8'. trachea 9. esophagus 10. fundus 11. body
12. pylorus 13. lesser curvature 14. greater curvature
15. duodenum

Photograph of the stomach shows two layers of the muscularis: the outer-longitudinal and inner-circular muscle layers. In addition to these, there is innermost oblique layer which is insufficiently developed, thus this can be seen only in the fundus and body portions. In the pyloric portion the well-developed circular muscles form the sphincter.

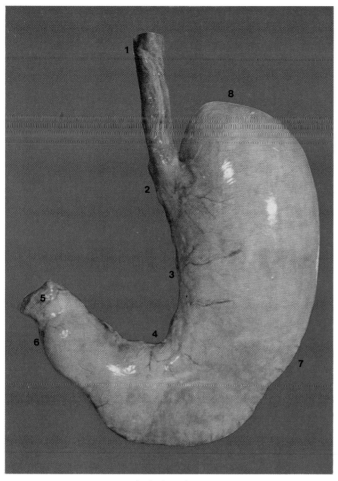

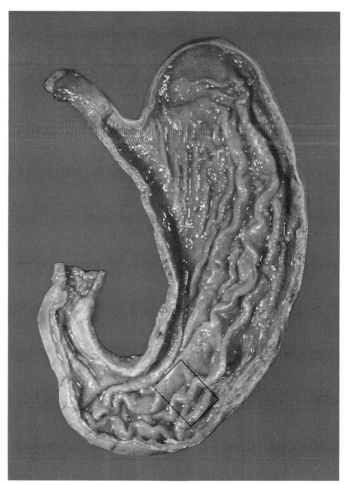

Anterior view

1. esophagus 2. cardia 3. lesser curvature 4. angular notch
5. duodenum 6. pylorus 7. greater curvature 8. fundus

Longitudinal section (interior)

The shape of the stomach is different in life and after death. The stomach in life presents a contracted shadatonic. In order to obtain a shadow in an X-ray examination, the patient is administered a radio-opaque material. Even the folds of the mucous membrane can be radiographed if the contrast material is applied properly. Any disorder in the fold is taken into account in diagnosing cancer or ulcer, etc.

The surface of the stomach is smooth, as it is covered by serosa (peritoneum). This is to ensure free movement of the stomach for digestion.

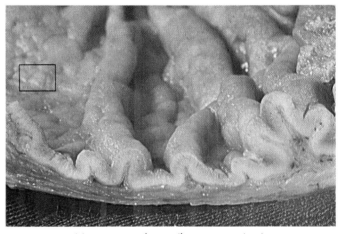

Mucous membrane (low-power view)

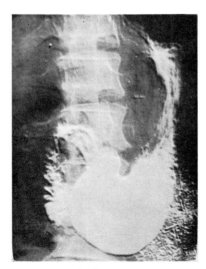

X-ray of the human stomach

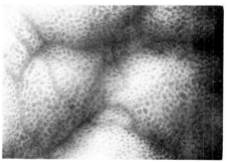

Mucous membrane (high-power view)

Small dots are the gastric pits (opening of the gastric glands).

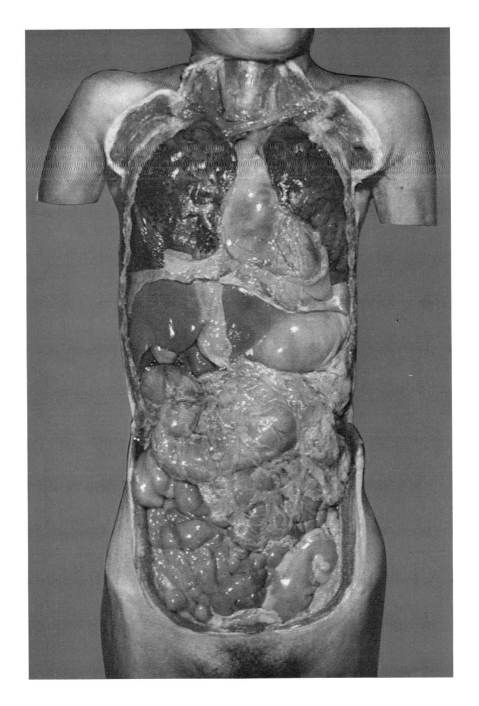

THORACIC and ABDOMINAL VISCERA

The photograph shows viscera of the thoracoabdominal section with the thoracic and abdominal walls removed. The diaphragm is cut at the anterior origin. Both ends of the stomach are hidden behind the diaphragm and the liver. The cecum is also veiled by the small intestine. The thin membranous caul hangs down anterior to the small intestine to protect the latter from rubbing against the abdominal wall.

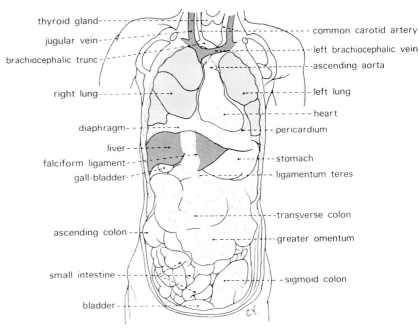

thyroid gland - - - - - - - - - common carotid artery
jugular vein - - - - - - - - - left brachiocephalic vein
brachiocephalic trunc - - - - - - - ascending aorta
right lung - - - - - - - - - left lung
- - - - - - - - - heart
diaphragm - - - - - - - - pericardium
liver - - - - - - - - -
falciform ligament - - - - - - - stomach
gall-bladder - - - - - - - - ligamentum teres
- - - - - - - - transverse colon
ascending colon - - - - - - - greater omentum
small intestine - - - - - - - - sigmoid colon
bladder - - - - - - - -

33

THE LENGTH OF THE DIGESTIVE TRACT

(as compared with the height of the human body)

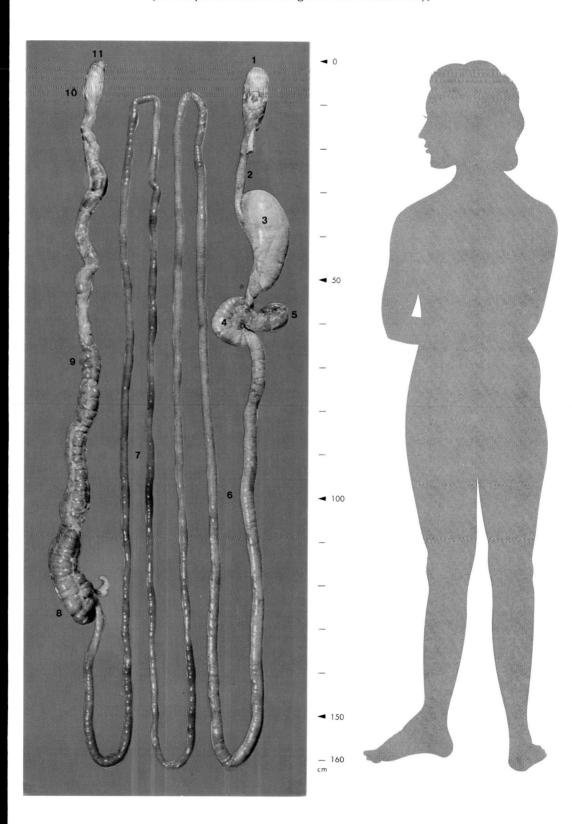

The small intestine starts at the duodenum (it derives its name from the fact that its length equals the width of twelve fingers) and runs down through the jejunum (meaning emptiness, which is in most cases the post-mortem state of this organ) and ileum (meaning an entangled or winding state) until it reaches the cecum. The large intestine starts from the cecum (meaning blind end), passes through the ascending, transverse, descending, and sigmoid colons into the rectum. The distended portion of the rectum slightly above the anus is referred to as the ampulla where the excreta is amassed.

1. tongue   2. esophagus   3. stomach   4. duodenum   5. pancreas   6. jejunum
7. ileum   8. cecum and appendix   9. colon   10. rectum   11. anus

DISPOSITION OF DIGESTIVE ORGANS

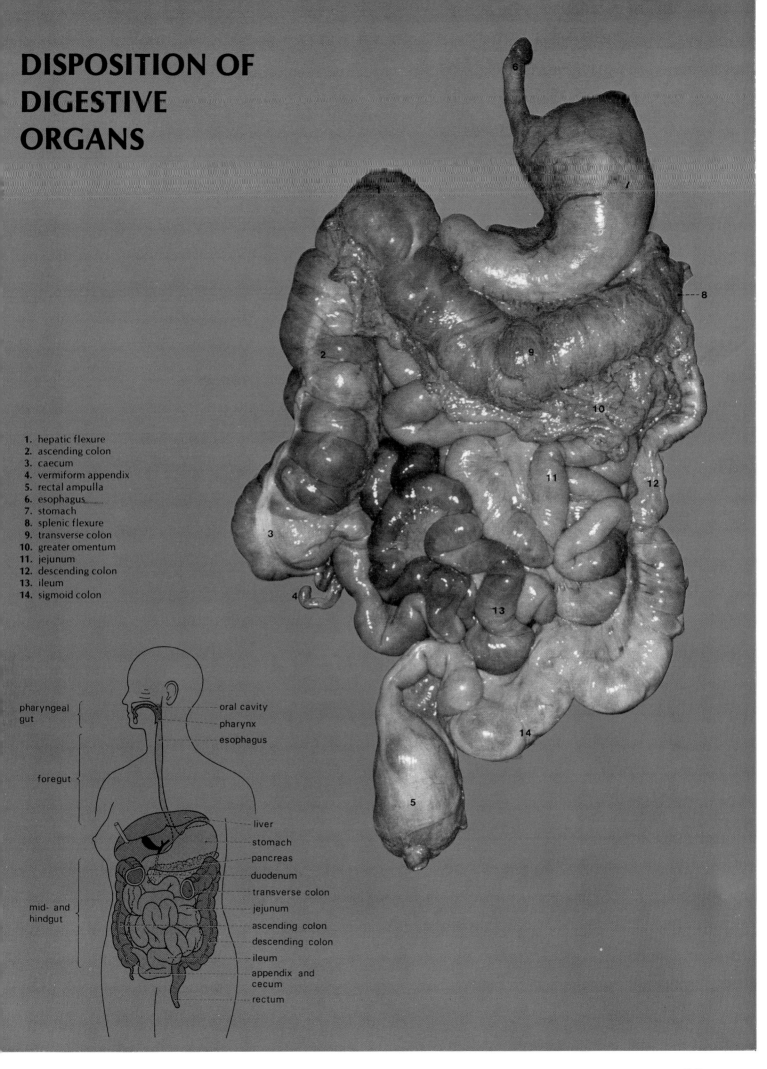

1. hepatic flexure
2. ascending colon
3. caecum
4. vermiform appendix
5. rectal ampulla
6. esophagus
7. stomach
8. splenic flexure
9. transverse colon
10. greater omentum
11. jejunum
12. descending colon
13. ileum
14. sigmoid colon

pharyngeal gut
oral cavity
pharynx
esophagus

foregut

liver
stomach
pancreas
duodenum
transverse colon
jejunum
ascending colon
descending colon
ileum
appendix and cecum
rectum

mid- and hindgut

COMPARISON OF THE VARIOUS SECTIONS OF THE INTESTINE

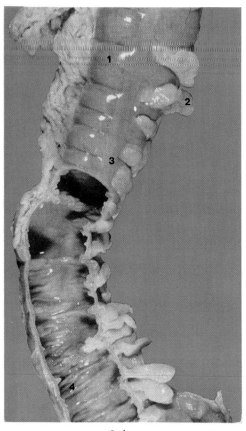

Colon

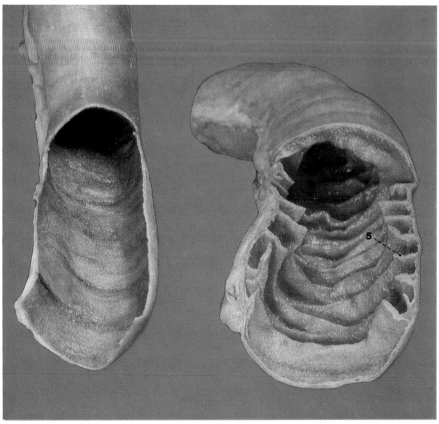

Ileum

Jejunum

The small intestine is divided into the jejunum (the upper two-fifths) and ileum (the lower three-fifths) although they are indistinguishable externally. Internally, however, the mucous membrane of the jejunum has distinct circular plica, while those of the ileum are obscure. The ileum has a characteristic lymphoid tissue (Peyer's patch). Along the exterior side of the colon are the tenia coli running longitudinally, as well as the epiploic appendages. There are also three corresponding plica on the mucous membrane.

1. haustra **2.** epiploic appendage **3.** tenia **4.** semilunar plica **5.** circular plica **6.** ascending colon **7.** cecum **8.** vermiform appendix **9.** mesenteriole **10.** ileum

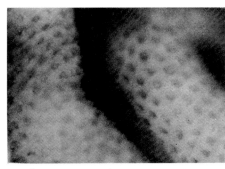

High power view of mucous membrane of the large intestine.

Instead of villi the large intestine has simple, tubular glands (crypts) and secretes large amounts of mucus which helps the passage of hard clods of feces.

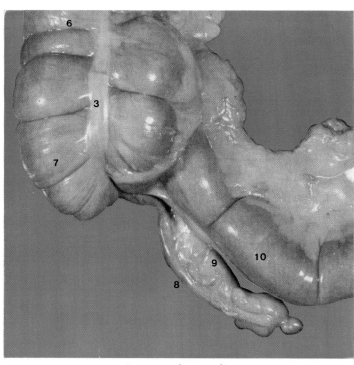

Cecum and appendix

36

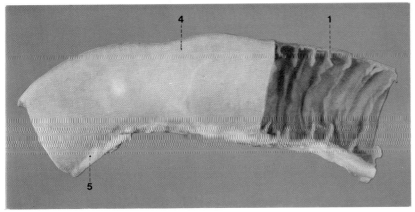

Exterior aspect of the jejunum and its mucous membrane

1. circular fold
2. circular muscle
3. longitudinal muscle
4. serous coat
5. mesentery

The mucous membrane of the duodenum is covered by the protuberant circular folds, which serve to increase the surface area of the membrane. Descending from the jejunum to the ileum, these folds gradually become inconspicuous. The ileum is characterized by the lymphoid tissue shown right below.

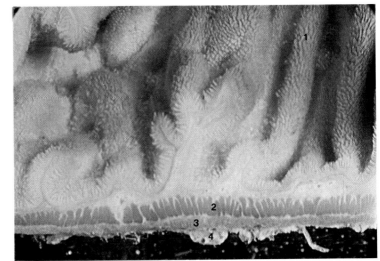

Mucous membrane with villi (enlarged)

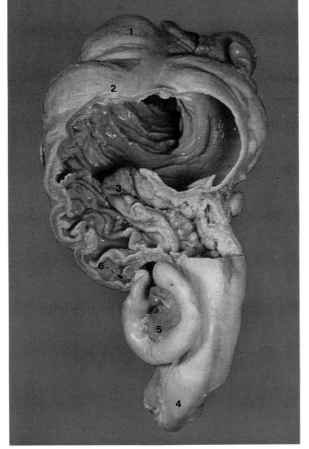

Cecum and appendix

1. ascending colon
2. cecum
3. ileocecal valve
   (upper and lower lips)
4. ileum
5. vermiform process
   (appendix)
6. orifice of appendix

At the junction of the ileum and cecum, there is the ileocecal valve, which prevents backward flow of dirty contents into the large intestine. At the end of cecum, there is the vermiform process or appendix, which is approximately 5—6 cm in length. This has large collections of lymphoid tissue, which occasionally become the source of inflammation.

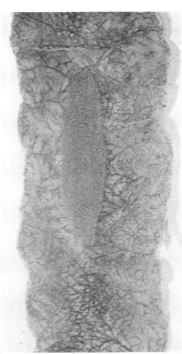

Aggregated lymphatic nodule
(Peyer's patch)
Aggregated lymphatic nodule found only in ileum, when affected by tubercle or typhoid bacilli, form an ulcer and sometimes cause perforation.

LIVER

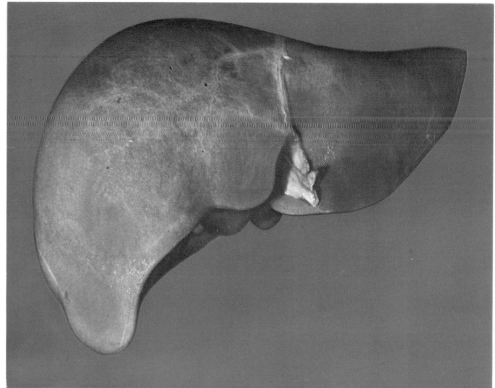

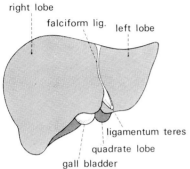

right lobe
falciform lig.
left lobe
ligamentum teres
quadrate lobe
gall bladder

Anterior aspect of the liver

The liver is the largest solid organ in the human body, weighing approximately 1,200 gr. Since the upper posterior surface adheres to the diaphragm, the entire liver moves vertically during respiration. The liver secretes bile and accumulates glycogen absorbed by the small intestine, in addition to its function of detoxifying injurious substances by dissolving them. The bile is collected temporarily in the gall bladder through the cystic duct, and is preserved in a concentrated state. It is secreted together with the pancreatic juice into the duodenum when food is channelled through it. Round ligament in the falciform ligament of the liver shown above is a obliterated umbilical vein which is the channel for blood returning from the placenta at the embryonic stage (cf. p. 75).

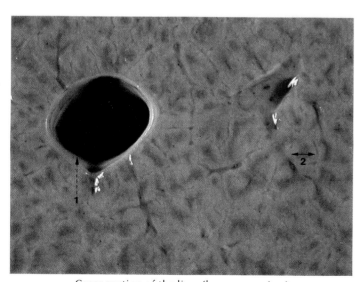

Cross-section of the liver (low-power view)
1. vein (about 8 mm in diameter)   **2.** lobule

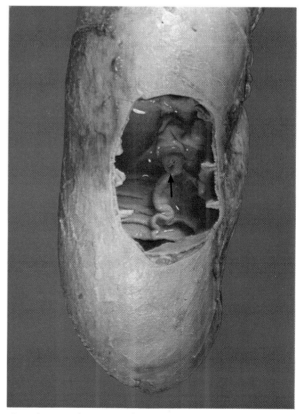

Duodenum (fenestrated to show the opening of bile and pancreatic ducts — (↑) duodenal papilla)

PANCREAS

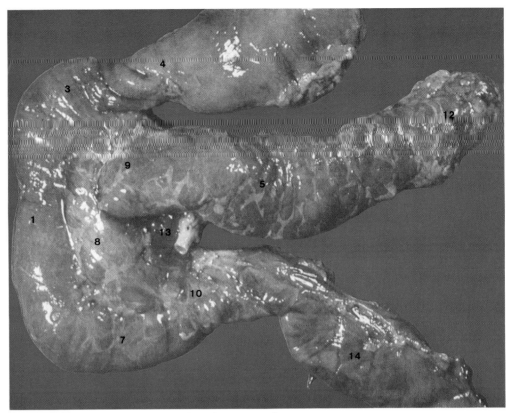

Anterior aspect of pancreas

The pancreas, which is located behind the stomach extending obliquely upward to the left, produces pancreatic juice (digestive juice) and insulin (hormone). The latter is produced in the islets of Langerhans, but is invisible macroscopically (about 0.1 —0.2 mm in diameter).

1. descending part (duodenum) **2.** common bile duct **3.** superior part (d.)
4. pylorus (stomach) **5.** body (pancreas) **6.** opening of main pancreatic ducts **6′.** accessory pancreatic duct (Santorini) **7.** horizontal part (d.)
8. uncinate process (p.) **9.** head (p.) **10.** ascending part (d.) **11.** pancreatic duct (Wirsung) **12.** tail (p.) **13.** superior mesenteric artery and vein
14. jejunum

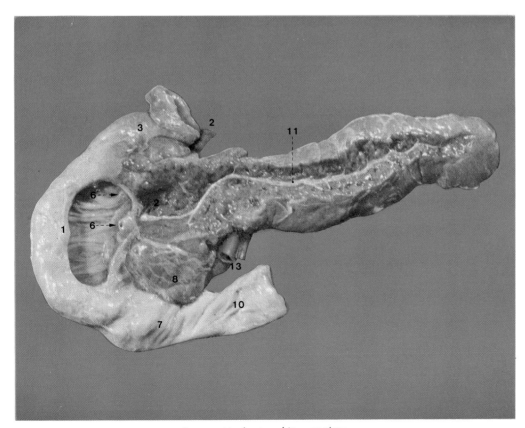

Pancreatic duct and its opening

NASAL
CAVITY

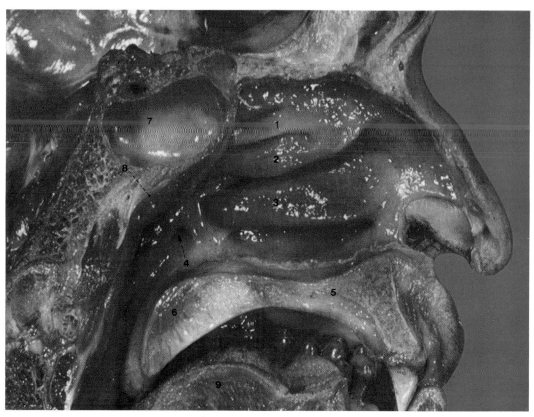

Lateral wall (the nasal septum is removed)

1. superior concha 2. middle concha 3. inferior concha 4. eustachian tube opening 5. hard palate
6. soft palate 7. sphenoidal sinus 8. nasopharyngeal tonsil 9. tongue 10. nasal septum 11. frontal
sinus 12. medulla oblongata 13. vocal ligament (vocal fold) 14. trachea 15. esophagus 16. spinal
cord 17. epiglottis

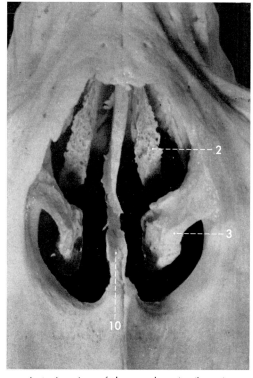

Anterior view of the nasal cavity (bone)

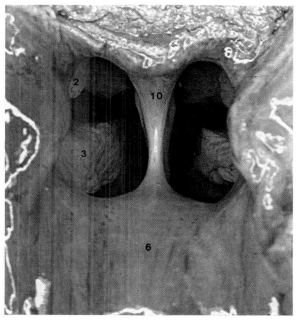

Posterior view of the nasal cavity (choanae)

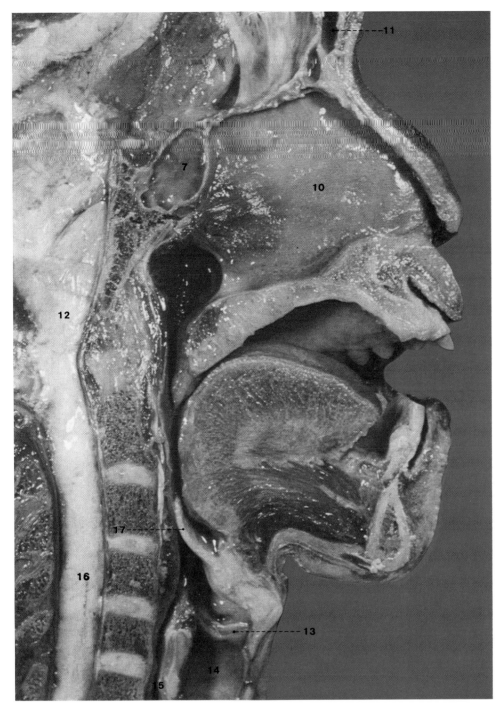

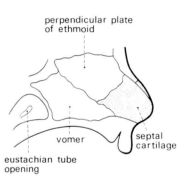

perpendicular plate
of ethmoid

vomer

septal
cartilage

eustachian tube
opening

Nasal septum

The nasal septum, which divides the nasal cavity at its center, is composed of two bones and cartilage. The interior of the cavity is quite spacious and there are three nasal conchae, superior, middle and inferior, which provide the nasal cavity with more surface area and also function as radiators by adjusting the temperature and humidity of the air inhaled. The superior nasal concha and the mucous membrane in the corresponding part of the nasal septum, which together make up the olfactory mucosa, have the function of scenting odors. The mucous membrane of the superior concha and adjacent part of the septum appears dull yellow, named olfactory area.

The opening of the eustachian tube is the mouth of the tube connecting the tympanic and nasal cavities, by means of which the air pressure within the tympanic cavity and that exterior to the tympanic membrane are balanced. When this tube is closed, it will affect hearing, since the vibration of the membrane is obstructed. (cf. p. 94)

LARYNX

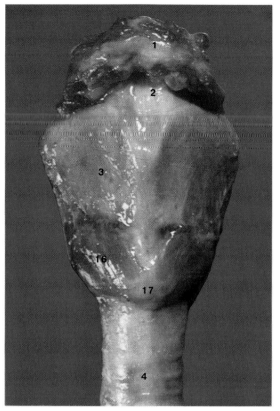

Anterior view

The vocal folds extend between the thyroid and arytenoid cartilages. The folds consist of the vocal muscle and vocal ligament. The long, narrow aperture between the vocal folds is called the glottis. During breathing, it opens wide, while during phonation, it narrows. The breath forced through this narrowed opening causes the rim of the vocal fold to vibrate, and thus creates voice. Just above the vocal fold is another similar fold referred to as the ventricular fold. It does not have any function in phonation, but is thought to be instrumental in maintaining moisture of the vocal folds.

At puberty, the male thyroid cartilage develops rapidly, causing the so-called change of voice. In the female, however, this vocal change is not as pronounced, since the whole larynx is small.

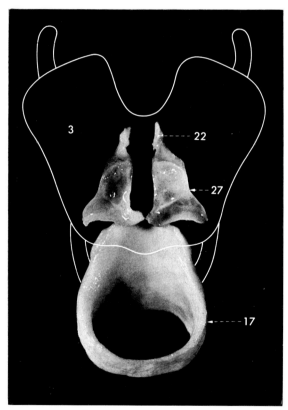

Cartilages of larynx (anterior view)

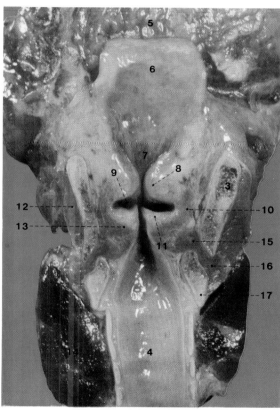

Frontal section (posterior view)

1. hyoid bone
2. thyrohyoid membrane
3. thyroid cartilage
4. trachea
5. tongue
6. epiglottis
7. vestibule
8. vestibular (ventricular) fold
9. ventricle
10. thro-arytenoid m.

11. vocal fold
12. thro-hyoid m.
    sterno-hyoid m.
    inf. constrictor
13. vocal m.
14. thyroid gland
15. lat. crico-arytenoid m.
15'. post. crico-arytenoid m.
16. crico-thyroid m.
17. cricoid cartilage

18. med. glossoepiglottic fold
19. vallecula
20. glottis
21. cuneiform cartilage
22. corniculate cartilage
23. pharynx
24. oblique arytenoid m.
25. transverse arytenoid m.
26. piriform recess
27. arytenoid cartilage

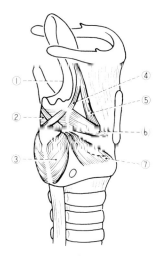

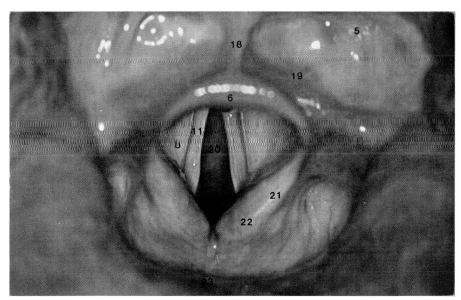

1. aryepiglottic plica　**2.** arytenoid muscle　**3.** post. cricoarytenoid m. **4.** aryepiglottic m.　**5.** thyroepiglottic m. **6.** thyroarytenoid m.　**7.** lat. arytenoid m.

Glottis (superior view)

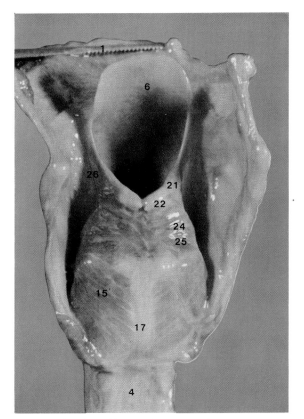

Muscles of larynx (posterior view)

The epiglottis projects like a screen, which is able to flap backward by swallowing foods and drinks to prevent them from entering into the trachea.

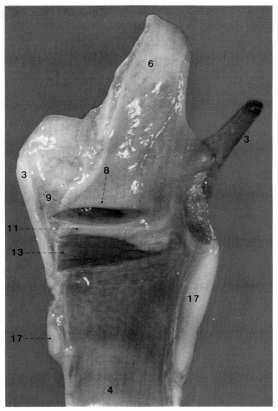

anterior　　Sagittal section　　posterior

Mucous membrane has been removed to show vocal ligaments and vocal muscle.

TRACHEA and BRONCHIAL TREE

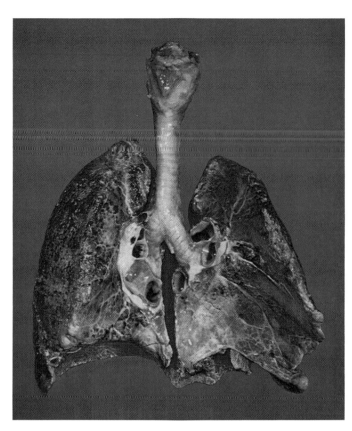

The trachea bifurcates into two extrapulmonary bronchi. Then they are further divided into intrapulmonary bronchi. As they branch, the intrapulmonary bronchi become progressively smaller in diameter and become bronchioles and finally reach the alveolar sac.

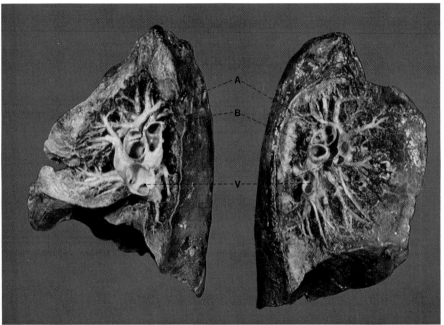

A. pulmonary artery   B. bronchus   V. pulmonary vein

Hilus of the lung

The heart is removed. The trachea is divided into the left and right bronchi. The section leading to the lung is called the hilus, through which the blood vessels and nerves enter or leave the lung with the bronchi. The cross-sections are that of the pulmonary arteries and veins.

The wall of the trachea and of the bronchus has numerous horseshoe-formed cartilages which are arranged regularly. They are important for enduring the negative pressure caused by respiration. Since the dorsal part of the walls is devoid of the cartilage and is bridged by bundles of smooth muscle fibers, the diameter of the canal can be controlled and changed by this smooth muscle tissue. Many mucous glands are located in the subcutaneous layer. Mucus catches dust and is brought up as phlegm.

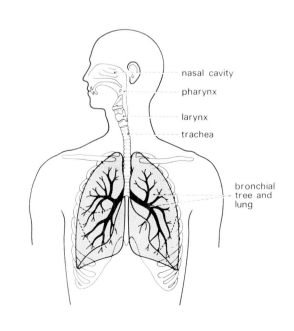

nasal cavity

pharynx

larynx

trachea

bronchial tree and lung

LUNGS

Lateral view

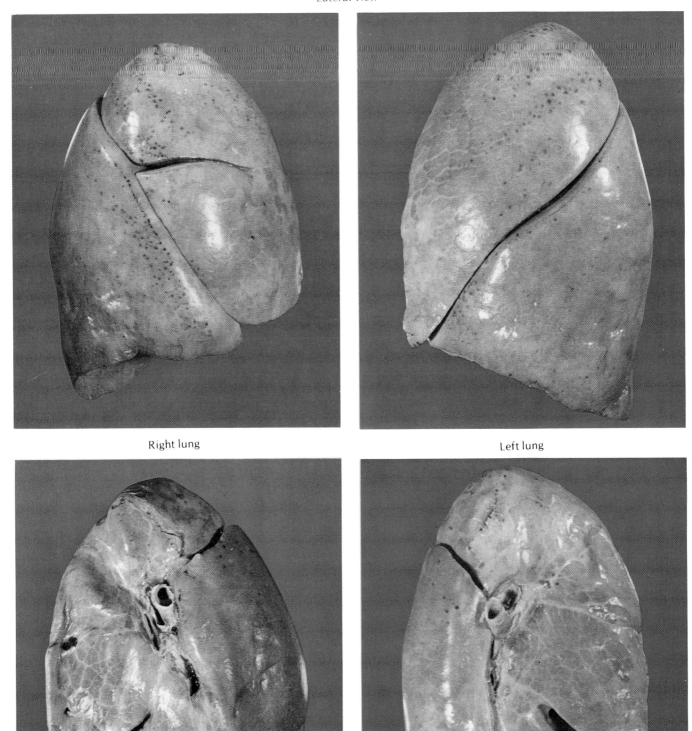

Right lung

Left lung

Medial (mediastinal) view

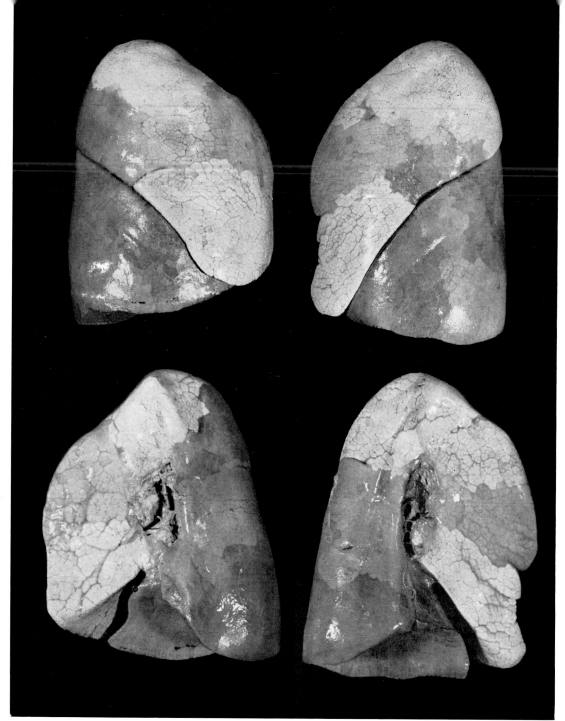

Bronchopulmonary Segments

The right lung is slightly larger than the left because of the position of the heart slightly to the left of the median line. The right lung consists of three lobes, while the left has only two. Each lobe is composed of pulmonary segments about 5 cm cube, ten in the right lung and nine in the left. The size and shape of the segments vary according to individuals. The lung in the upper photograph, which is rather exceptional, is somewhat different from those shown below, which are taken from a textbook.

Each of the pulmonary segments comprises slightly more than ten lobules, each of which is approximately 1.5 cm cube. These lobules, known as secondary lobules, further consist of several primary lobules, which in turn consist of countless alveoli (p. 47).

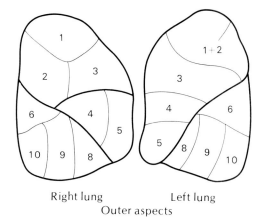

Right lung   Left lung
Outer aspects

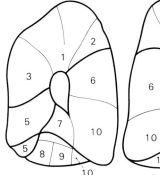
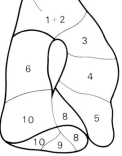

Right lung   Left lung
Inner aspects

Right lung
1. apical ⎫
2. posterior ⎬ superior lobe
3. anterior ⎭
4. lateral ⎫
5. medial ⎬ middle lobe

6. superior (apical) ⎫
7. medial basal ⎪
8. anterior basal ⎬ inferior lobe
9. lateral basal ⎪
10. posterior basal ⎭

Left lung
1. apicoposterior ⎫
2. anterior ⎪
3. superior lingular ⎬ superior lobe
4. inferior lingular ⎭

5. superior (apical) ⎫
6. medial basal ⎪
8. anterior-medial basal ⎬ inferior lobe
9. lateral basal ⎪
10. posterior basal ⎭

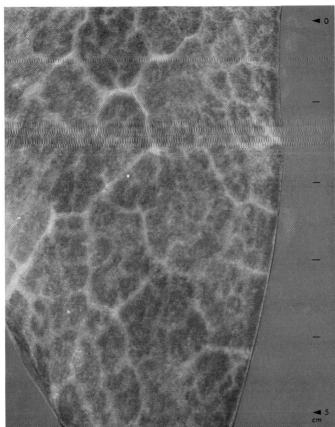

A typical clean lung

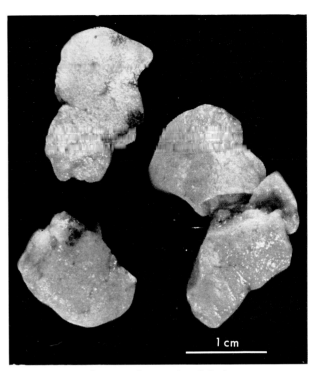

Separated secondary lobule

As each segment has its exclusive bronchus and blood supply, it is resected in units of the segment in surgical operations, for example in case of tuberculosis.

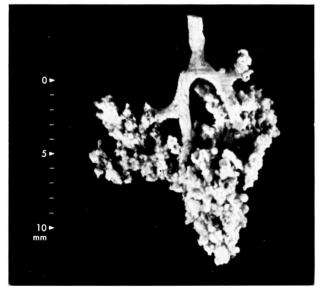

Cast alveolus
An alveolus is a small bag, open on the side which faces the respiratory bronchiole. The small globes are the alveolar sacks.

a. epiglottis **b.** thyroid cartilage **c.** trachea
d. right main bronchus **e.** bifurcation **f.** left main bronchus
(*cf.* p. 46: No. 1 — 10)

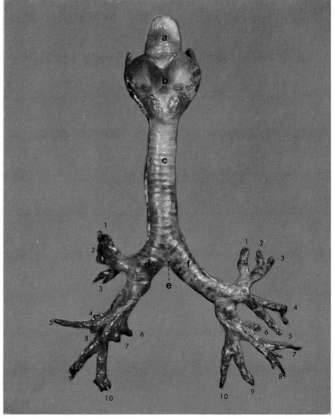

Anterior aspect of larynx, trachea and bronchi

DIAPHRAGM

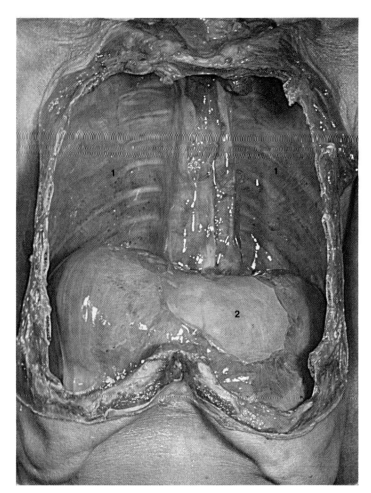

The diaphragm is a dome-shaped musculo-fibrous septum which separates the thoracic from the abdominal cavity. Its peripheral parts attach to the sternum, ribs, and the anterior parts of the upper lumbar vertebrae. The central part lacking muscle fibers directly fuses with the pericardium. The diaphragm is penetrated by three canals; aorta, esophagus and inferior vena cava.

1. thoracic wall covered with pleura
2. pericardial sack
3. lung
4. heart
5. central tendon
6. inf. vena cava
7. esophagus
8. aorta
9. lumber part
10. right crus
11. quadratus lumborum
12. psoas
13. iliacus
14. lumbar vertebrae
15. rectum
16. uterus and adnexa
17. transversus abd. m.
18. spinal cord

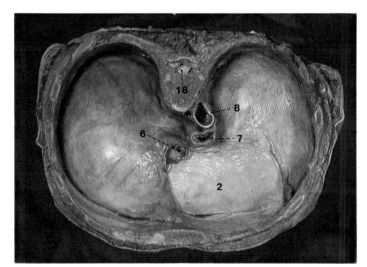

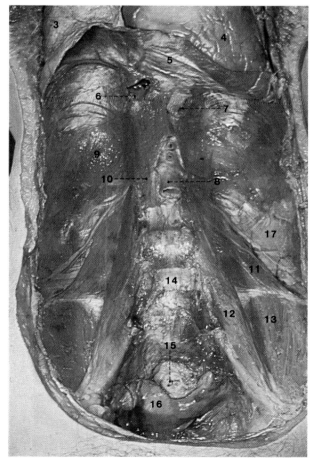

KIDNEY

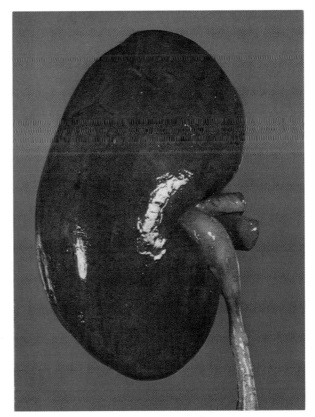
Dorsal view (left kidney)

The kidney is a bean-shaped organ about 10 cm. in length longitudinally. Its section reveals the cortex, medulla and renal pelvis in the center. The cortex consists of the renal corpuscle and convoluted tubule surrounding it. The medulla is composed of longitudinal ducts (Henle's loop and collecting duct) which are distinguishable with the naked eye. The medullary substance forms pyramids tipped by papillae, between which the cortical substance bulges to form columns. The pelvis of the kidney serves only as a place for collecting urine. Because of the kidney's function of extruding waste matters generated in the body, the renal vessels are disproportionately large.

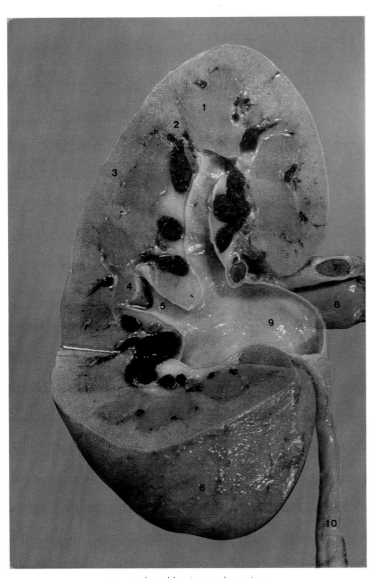
Frontal and horizontal section

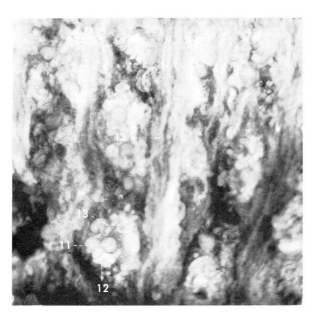
Nephrons and collecting tubules
(highly magnified)

1. renal pyramid   2. renal column   3. cortex
4. papilla   5. minor calyx   6. fibrous capsule
7. renal artery   8. renal vein   9. renal pelvis
10. ureter   11. renal corpuscle   12. proximal
convoluted tubules   13. distal convoluted tubules
14. collecting tubules

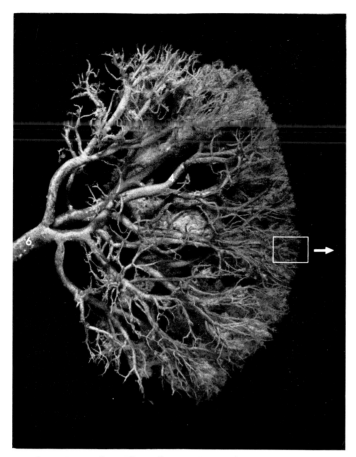

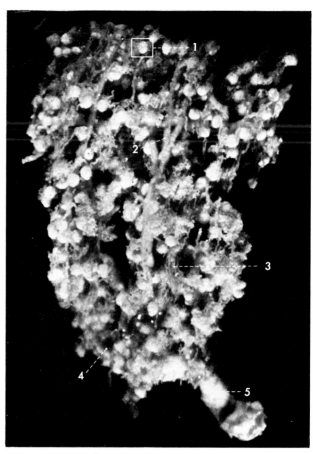

Cast of renal artery (natural size)

Cast of renal artery (low power view)

1. glomerulus 2. interlobular artery 3. capillary loops 4. interlobar artery 5. arcuate artery 6. renal artery

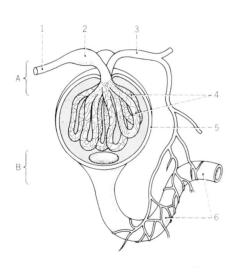

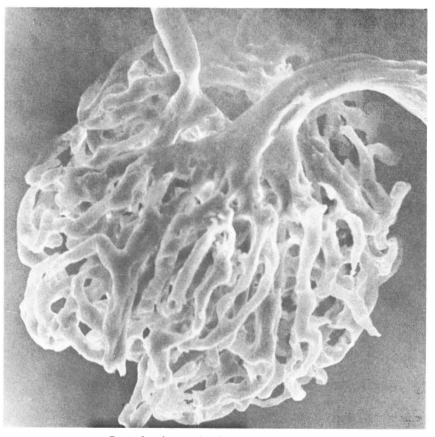

A. Vascular pole B. Urinary pole 1. afferent arteriole 2. pole cushion 3. efferent arteriole 4. glomerulus with podocytes 5. Bowman's capsule 6. uriniferous tubules (proximal convoluted tubule)

Cast of a glomerulus (high power view)

COMPLETE VIEW OF THE UROGENITAL SYSTEM

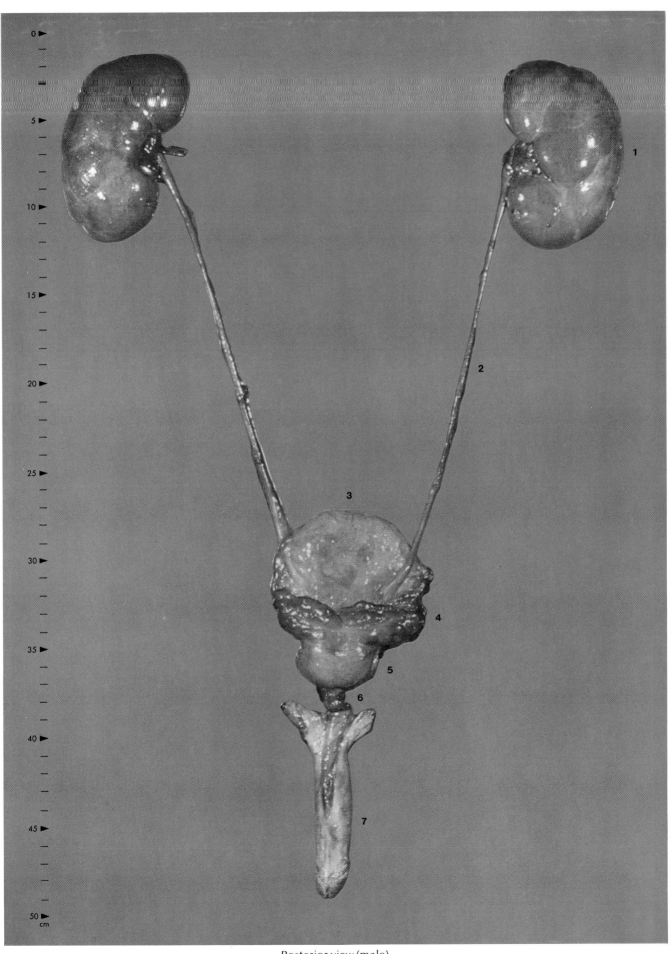

Posterior view (male)

1. kidney   2. ureter   3. bladder   4. seminal vesicle   5. prostate   6. urethra and Cowper's gland   7. penis

BLADDER

These two photographs are on the same reduced scale.

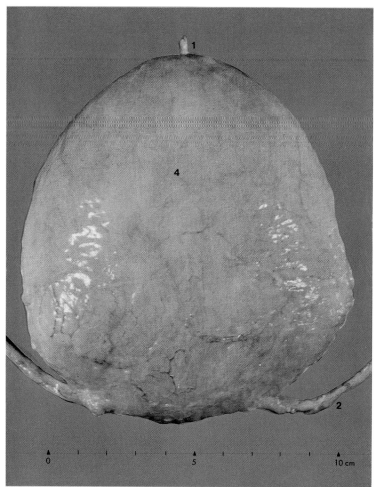

Posterior view (female), 300 ml

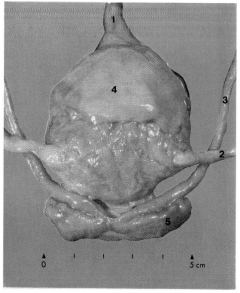

Posterior view (male), empty

1. median umbilical ligament
2. ureter **3.** ductus deferens
4. peritoneum **5.** vesicula seminalis
6. orifice of ureter **7.** urethra

Urine collected in the renal pelvis is carried by the peristaltic motion of the ureteral wall into the bladder. The bladder wall consists of three thick muscular layers and is highly distensible. When empty, it is about 1 cm thick (cf. p. 60) but when filled to capacity, it becomes diaphanously thin. Its normal capacity is about 470 ml in the male, and that of the female bladder is said to be five-sixths of man's. In the distended state, the bladder reaches about 5 cm above the symphysis.

Two ureters enter the posterior inferior wall of the bladder obliquely and this causes the anterior walls of the ureters to be pressed when the bladder is filled with urine, thus serving as valves to prevent the urine from flowing back upwards.

The two ureters and a urethra form a triangular area (urethral trigone) which retains the same dimensions whether the bladder is distended or contracted.

In the empty state, the bladder wall is thick with numerous wrinkles visible on the mucous membrane.

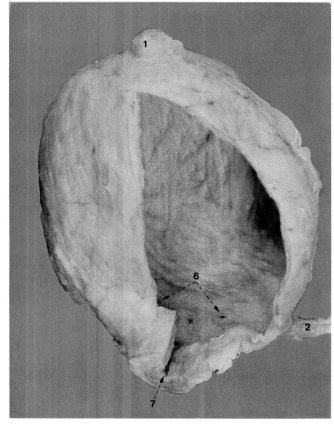

Trigonum vesicae*
Anterolateral view (female), empty

MALE GENITAL ORGANS

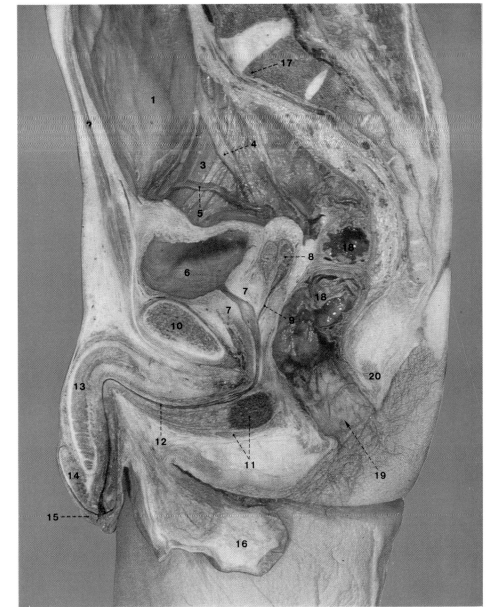

Meidan sagittal section of male pelvis (the pelvic peritoneum removed.)

1. abdominal cavity proper
2. rectus abdominis
3. psoas
4. ureter
5. ductus deferens
6. urinary bladder
7. prostate
8. seminal vesicle
9. ejaculatory duct
10. pubic symphysis
11. corpus spongiosum and bulbospongiosus muscle
12. urethra
13. corpus cavernosum
14. glans penis
15. prepuce
16. scrotum
17. promontry of sacrum
18. rectum
19. anus
20. sphincter ani externus

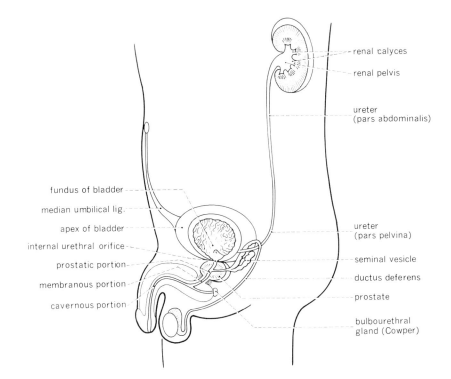

- renal calyces
- renal pelvis
- ureter (pars abdominalis)
- ureter (pars pelvina)
- seminal vesicle
- ductus deferens
- prostate
- bulbourethral gland (Cowper)

fundus of bladder
median umbilical lig.
apex of bladder
internal urethral orifice
prostatic portion
membranous portion
cavernous portion

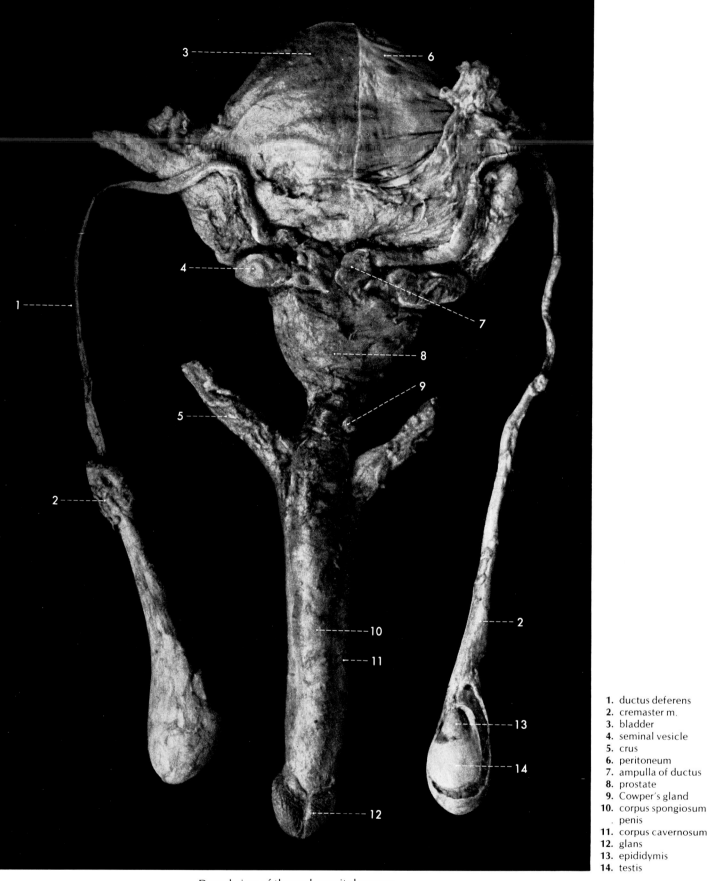

Dorsal view of the male genital organs

1. ductus deferens
2. cremaster m.
3. bladder
4. seminal vesicle
5. crus
6. peritoneum
7. ampulla of ductus
8. prostate
9. Cowper's gland
10. corpus spongiosum penis
11. corpus cavernosum
12. glans
13. epididymis
14. testis

Sperm generated in the testis pass through the epididymis and ductus deferens into the urethra where they mingle with a secretion of the prostate before they are ejaculated as semen. Seminal vesicles are located a little above the point where ductus deferens unite with the urethra and contribute a secretion to the seminal fluid. The bulbo-urethral (Cowper's) gland directly underneath the prostate secretes a colorless, transparent and viscous fluid which serves as a lubricant to the urethral meatus before coition.

Penis and Testis

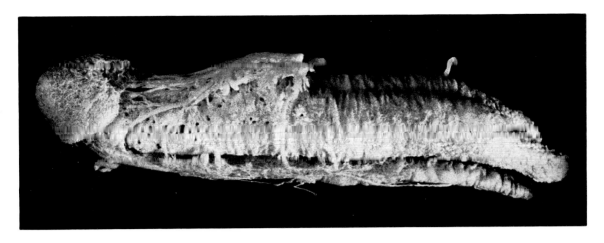

Cast of the erectile tissue: The penis consists of three cavernous bodies, which cause erection of the penis when suffused with blood. In this cast, resin has been injected. (*cf.* p. 60)

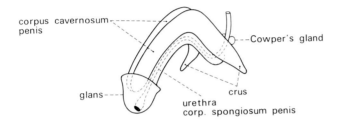

corpus cavernosum penis

Cowper's gland

glans

crus

urethra
corp. spongiosum penis

The testis is a mass of numerous seminiferous tubules, in which sperm is produced. The epididymis, it may be seen, also consists of a duct about 6 meters long, exceedingly convoluted, and is a store room for sperm.

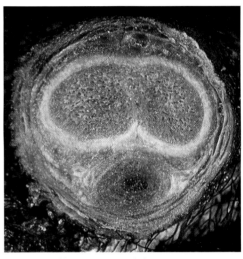

Cross-section of the penis

A. epididymis
B. testis

1. spermatic cord
2. tunica vaginalis (parietal layer)
3. gubernaculum
4. septum
5. lobule
6. tunica vaginalis (visceral layer)

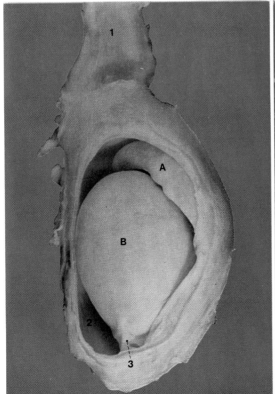

Testis, epididymis and their covering

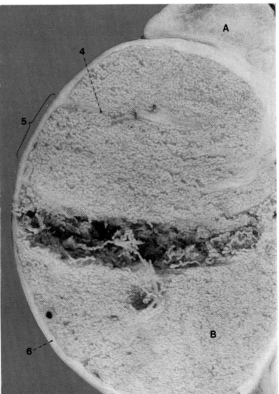

Seminiferous tubules longitudinal section

55

FEMALE GENITAL ORGANS

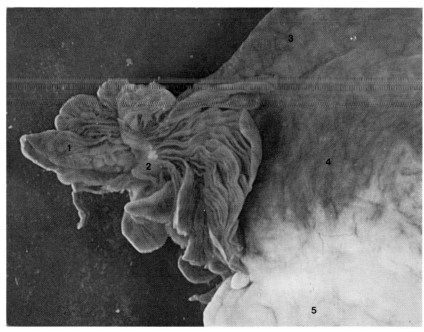

Fallopian tube and fimbria

Fallopian Tube and Ovary

1. fimbria **2.** abdominal ostium **3.** ampulla
4. mesosalpinx **5.** ovary

To show the opening of the Fallopian tube, yellow pigment was injected into the tube from the uterine opening.

The funnel-like end of the oviduct is known as the fimbria. An ovum is picked up by the fimbria which drapes over and clasps the surface of the ovary. The ovum cannot move of itself but is propelled to the uterus by the muscular action of the uterine tubes and by the movement of cilia lining the interior surface. Ovulation is followed by bleeding, which forms the corpus hemorrhagicum. This red body gradually turns into a yellow body (the corpus luteum). The luteal hormone activates uterine secretion to enable the ovum to attach itself to the wall of the uterus with greater ease.

After a certain period, the corpus luteum atrophies into the corpus albicans. Consequently the endometrium breaks down and menstruation takes place.

The total number of ova is said to be nearly 420,000 in embryo, and decrease after birth; only about 400 of these are ovulated in the course of a lifetime. Fertilization is considered to occur generally in the ampulla of the oviduct.

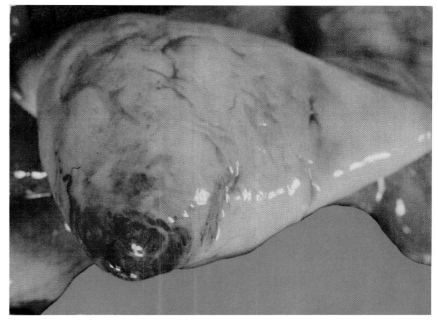

Ruptured follicle (corpus hemorrhagicum)

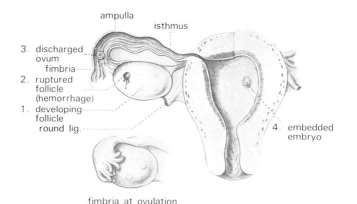

fimbria at ovulation

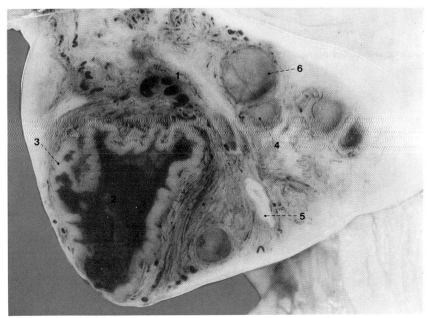

1. blood vessels **2.** corpus hemorrhagicum
3. corpus luteum   **4.** developing follicle
5. corpus albicans   **6.** Graafian follicle

Longitudinal section of ovary (*cf*. p. 56)

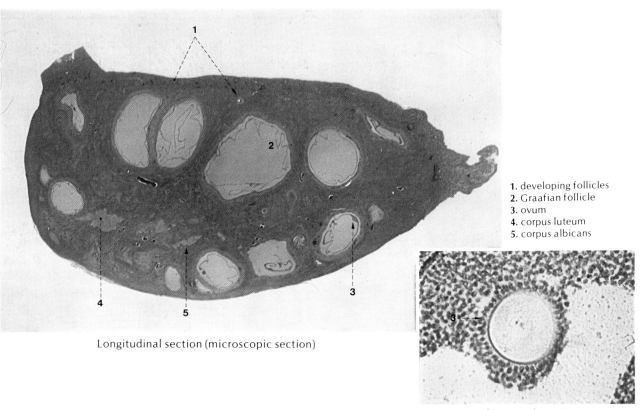

Longitudinal section (microscopic section)

1. developing follicles
2. Graafian follicle
3. ovum
4. corpus luteum
5. corpus albicans

Ovum (enlarged)

When a primordial follicle matures in the ovary, it fills with fluid to become a Graafian follicle. Though it grows to several millimeters in diameter, the ovum itself, which remains in a corner of the follicle, measures only a little more than 0.12 mm, In the course of time, the follicle matures and ruptures (ovulation), extruding the ovum. Then the follicle collapses and is transformed into the corpus luteum which secretes hormones that prepare the lining of the uterus for reception of the fertilized ovum and suppress consequent ovulation.

The hormones secreted from the follicle expedite the development of secondary sex characteristics.

Uterus and Adnexa

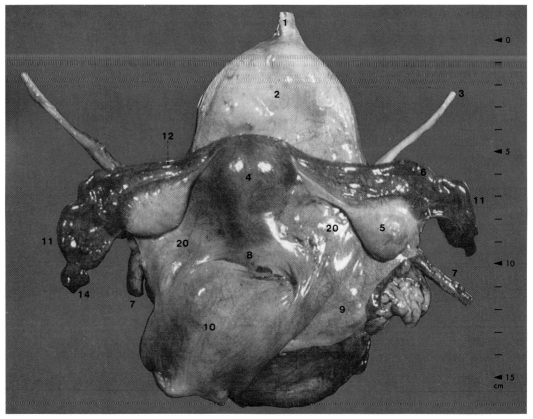

Dorsal view

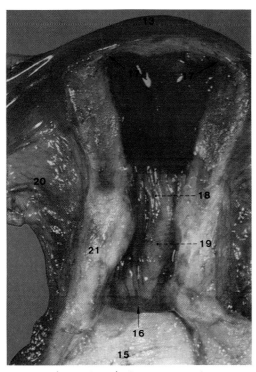

Endometrium during menstruation
(at the beginning stage)

1. median umbilical ligament
2. bladder
3. ureter
4. uterus
5. ovary
6. fallopian tube
7. round ligament
8. pouch of Douglas
9. peritoneum
10. rectum
11. ampulla tubae
12. isthmus tubae
13. fundus uteri
14. fimbria tubae
15. anterior wall of vagina

16. external os
17. ostium uterinum tubae
18. internal os
19. endocervical canal (palmate folds)
20. broad ligament
21. cervix uteri
22. glans clitoridis and prepuce
23. corpus clitoridis
24. crus clitoridis
25. labium minus
26. bulb of vestibule
27. greater vestibular gland
28. vaginal orifice
29. external urethral orifice

At the end of the premenstrual phase, the thickness of endometrium becomes maximal (about 5 mm) and it is congested with blood, then it falls off to be extruded with blood. The cervical canal of the uterus is plugged with extremely slimy mucus which prevents the invasion of microbes from outside.

58

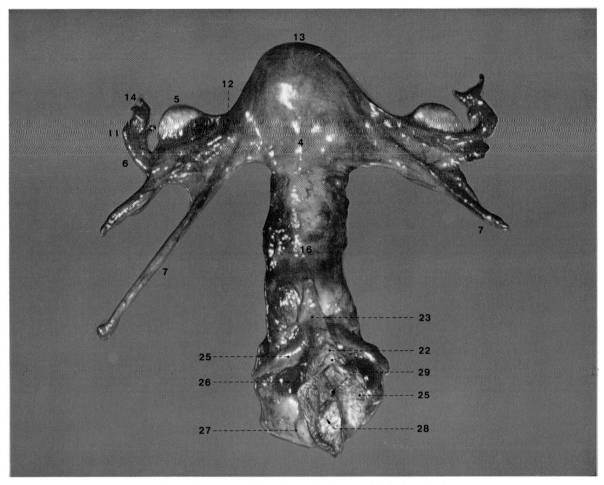

Complete view of female genital organs (Anterior view)

Uterus, Adnexa and External genitalia

Normally the uterus is bent forward because of the round ligaments (cf. p. 60). Sometimes, however, it assumes a backward position and is bent sharply backward due to the extended supporting ligaments. This phenomenon is known as retroflexion. In this position, nerves and blood vessels are drawn backwards, often resulting in lumbago and at times causing sterility. The round ligaments pass through the inguinal canal, traverse the superior edge of the pubic bone diagonally and terminate in the labium majus. By operation, the ligaments may be shortened to restore the normal position of the uterus. Although the inguinal canal is a natural aperture in the abdominal wall, it sometimes permits prolapse of the intestine, causing inguinal hernia. In the male body, the vas deferens runs through this canal.

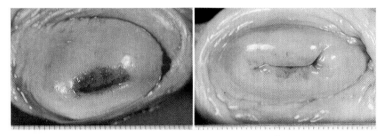

Nullipara   Multipara

External os of uterus (natural size)

The external orifice of the uterus distends at childbirth but contracts only to a certain degree. Inspection of the orifice, therefore, enables the doctor to distinguish nullipara from multipara readily.

59

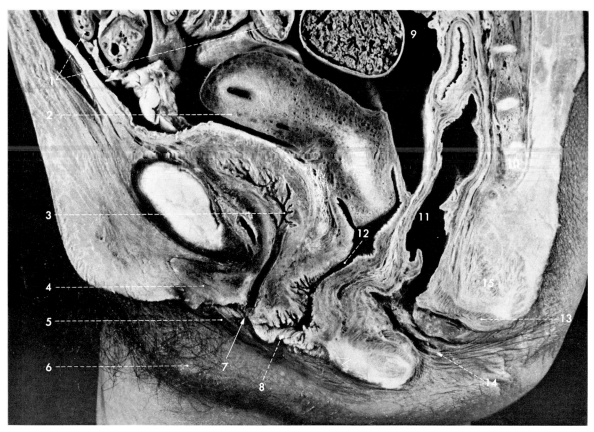

1.	small intestine
2.	uterus
3.	bladder (empty)
4.	clitoris
5.	labium minus
6.	labium majus
7.	urethra
8.	hymen
9.	sigmoid colon
10.	coccyx
11.	rectum
12.	vagina
13.	internal sphincter ani
14.	anus
15.	external sphincter ani

Midsagittal section of the female lumbar region (*virgin*)

This picture clearly shows the relative position of the bladder, uterus, vagina and rectum. Since it is completely empty, the bladder is markedly contracted and its wall is thick. The uterus is anteverted, but its position is affected by the collected amount of urine or feces. In many cases the uterus leans off the median line either to the right or the left. Therefore in this picture only part of the cavity is visible.

The vagina is about 7 cm in length, normally collapsed with the anterior and dorsal walls in contact. The vaginal wall has numerous transverse folds, which help to increase friction during coition. No secreting glands are present in the vaginal mucous membrane but it is moistened by a transudation through the epithelium with the addition of mucus from the uterus. The amount of fluid increases extremely in the state of erotism. There is no sensation of pain from the vagina to the external orifice of the uterus. The vaginal wall consists of smooth muscle, so it cannot contract voluntarily. Orgasm, however, causes contraction of the vaginal wall.

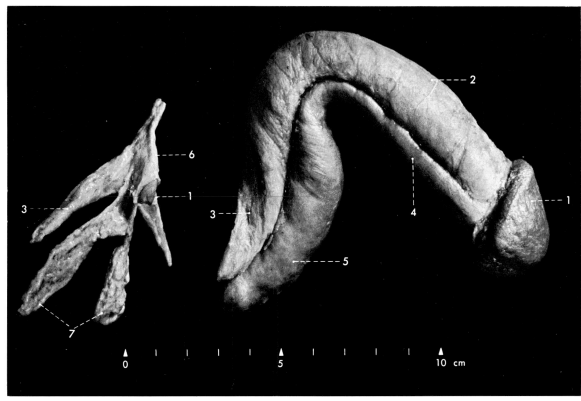

Comparison of clitoris (left) and penis (right)

Female External Genitalia

There exist considerable individual differences in the shape, thickness and extensibility of the hymen. Consequently it is not always possible to judge a woman's virginity by her hymen. Three typical cases of the hymen are introduced here.

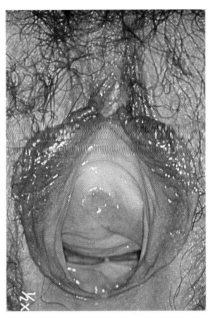

Hymen of multipara

In this case, the hymen disappeared, and the contact of anterior and posterior wall of vagina is observed. In most cases, the shrunken remnants of hymen are seen, and are called carunculae hymenales.

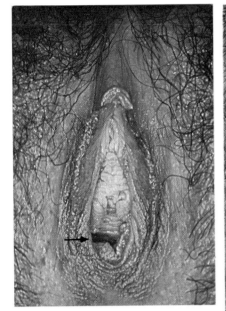

Ruptured hymen

The part indicated by the arrow is torn, but the question is whether it was a result of coition or not. Contrary to a common belief, however, the hymen cannot be torn by vigorous exercise.

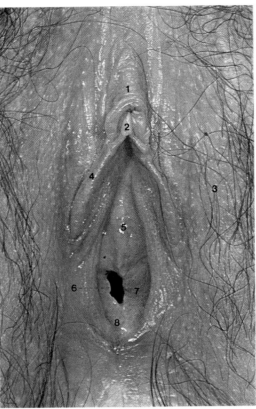

1. prepuce   2. clitoris (glans)
3. labium majus   4. labium minus
5. urethral orifice   6. vaginal orifice
7. hymen   8. vestibular fossa

Complete hymen (19 years old)

This hymen barely admitted one finger. It is only when the hymen is complete like this that a woman's virginity can be affirmed conclusively. The labium minus is small.

There are remarkable individual differences in the shape and size of labium minus. It abounds with pigment and has the appearance of mucous membrane. But it is actually skin (sweat and sebaceous glands exist).

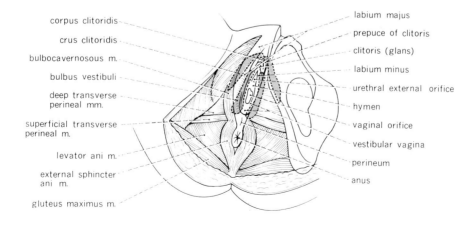

corpus clitoridis
crus clitoridis
bulbocavernosous m.
bulbus vestibuli
deep transverse perineal mm.
superficial transverse perineal m.
levator ani m.
external sphincter ani m.
gluteus maximus m.

labium majus
prepuce of clitoris
clitoris (glans)
labium minus
urethral external orifice
hymen
vaginal orifice
vestibular vagina
perineum
anus

1. glans   2. corpus cavernosum penis   3. crus   4. corpus spongiosum   5. bulb   6. body of clitoris   7. bulb of vestibule

Though different in size, the penis and the clitoris are homologues. Composed of cavernous bodies, both erect when they are filled with blood. Glans clitoridis is far smaller than glans penis, but the former is said to contain as many termini of sensory nerves as the latter. Because of this extremely high density of sensory nerve endings, glans clitoridis is far more sensitive than glans penis. Both clitoris and penis are securely attached to the inferior edge of the pubic bone, so they do not dangle when erection occurs.

GROWTH OF THE FETUS

Menstruation is suspended by fertilization. As birth occurs approximately 280 days after the beginning of the last menstrual period, months are counted in terms of 28 days. In the early stage of growth, the human fetus is nearly indistinguishable from that of other animals, the pig, for instance. Equipped with a tail, the human fetus attests to its animal origin. The fourth month witnesses an increasing humanization in the appearance of the embryo, but many days are still required before it reaches full growth. In the case of a male embryo, for instance, the testis does not reach into the scrotum until about the seventh month. Until then the scrotum is empty.

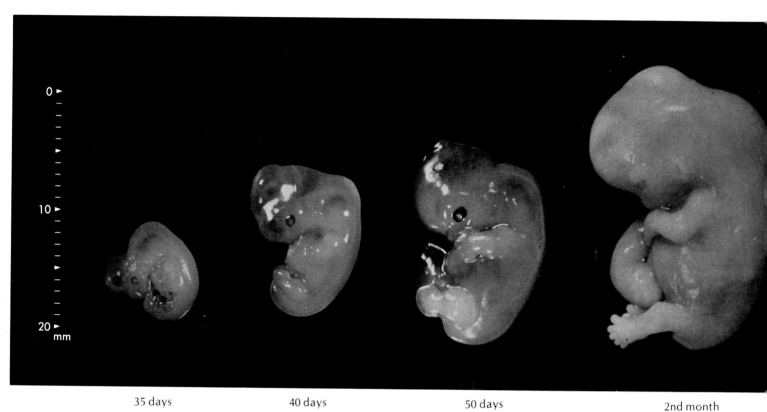

| 35 days | 40 days | 50 days | 2nd month |

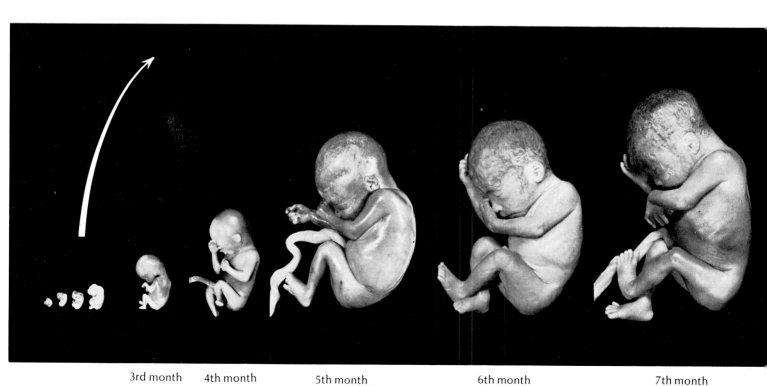

| 3rd month | 4th month | 5th month | 6th month | 7th month |

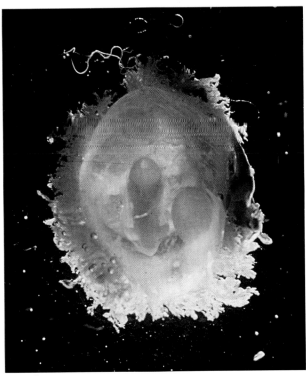

A photograph of the embryo in the chorionic sac
(about 5 mm length estimated age, 32 days)
A ball at the right is yolk sac.

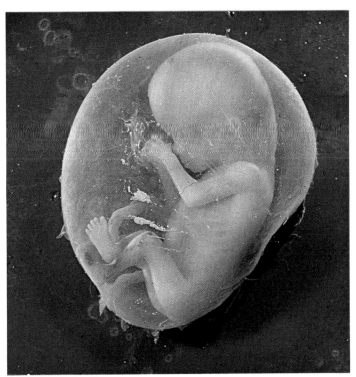

63 mm embryo (about 3rd month) in the amnion

The fetus is surrounded by the amnion, filled with amniotic fluid, so that the developing fetus is actually floating in a fluid environment. The rupture of the amnion and the outflow of the fluid is called amniorrhexis. As is shown in the picture, a baby may be born in the amniotic sac.

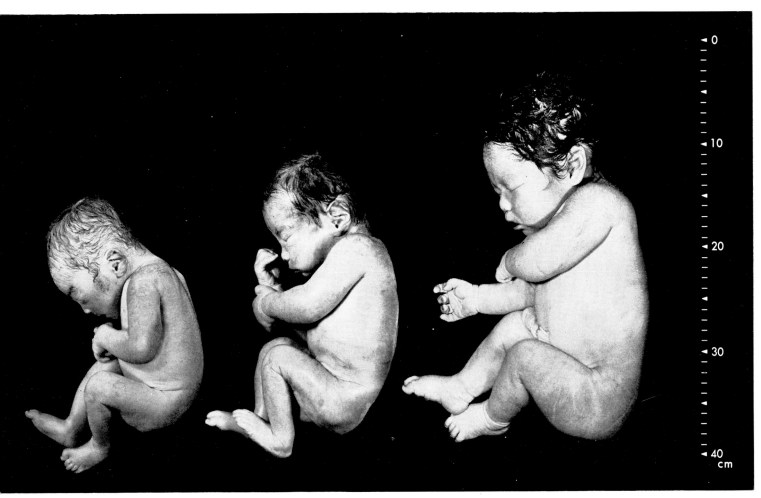

8th month   9th month   10th month of pregnancy

Uterus at Pregnancy

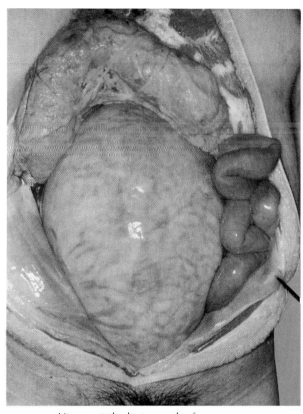

The uterus expands considerably with the growth of the fetus. Near birth the uterine wall is about 1 cm. thick and the weight is twenty to thirty times that of the normal uterus. The uterus contracts to normal size in six to ten weeks after birth. When pregnancy occurs, the external orifice of the uterus and vagina softens remarkably and increases extensibility in preparation for delivery.

Uterus at the last month of pregnancy

Placenta

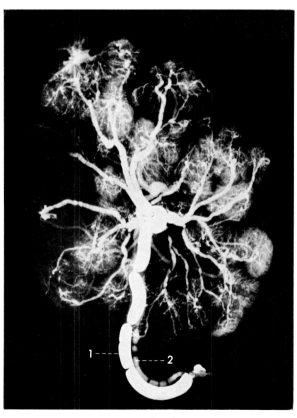

Some of the blood vessels in the umbilical cord, unlike those in our body, have sphincteral functions. The constricted part of the blood vessel in the picture illustrates this function. It prevents excessive bleeding when the umbilical cord is cut.

In the placenta, the umbilical artery breaks up into many branches. There is no continuity between the mother's blood and that of the fetus, which are separated by a thin membrane. Germs, however, sometimes penetrate this membrane to affect the fetus. Congenital syphilis is caused in this way.

Angiogram of a placenta
1. umbilical vena **2.** umbilical artery

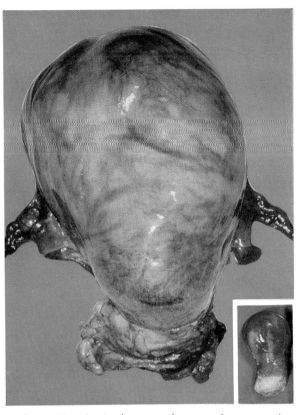

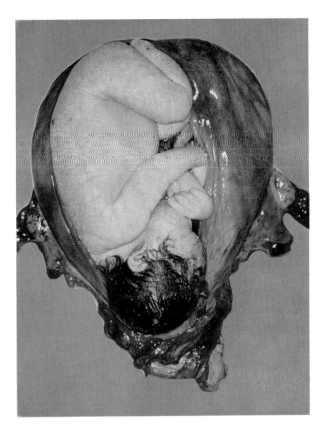

Comparison in size between the normal uterus and the uterus at pregnancy.
left: The uterus in the final stage of pregnancy.
right: The uterus in the normal state.

Fetus in uterus

The placenta is 15 to 20 cm in diameter, 2 to 3 cm in thickness and weighs 500 to 600 gm. The maternal aspect of it is lobulated.

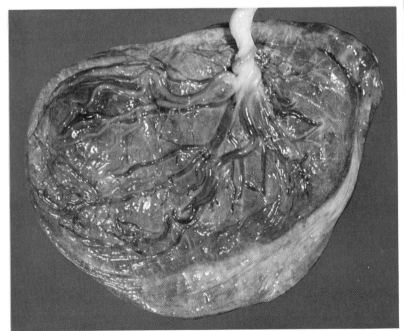

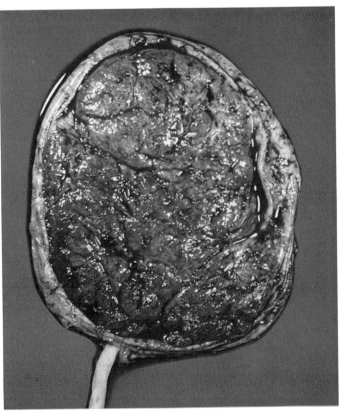

Placenta (fetal aspect; covered with amnion)
red: umbilical arteries   blue: umbilical vena

Placenta (maternal aspect)

ENDOCRINE ORGANS

Thyroid gland
Controls the metabolic rate of the body.

Parathyroid gland
Regulates salt, especially calcium metabolism

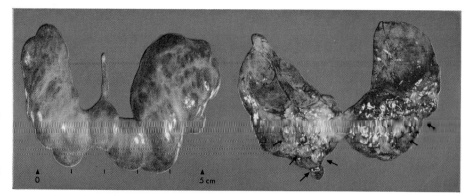

Thyroid gland (anterior view)　　　　(posterior view) and parathyroid gland (↑)

Suprarenal (adrenal) body
The cortex (corticosteroid etc.):
Controls salt and sugar metabolism and secretes sex hormones.
The medula (adrenaline):
Raises the blood pressure

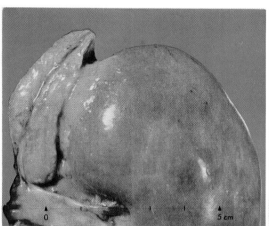

Kidney and suprarenal gland

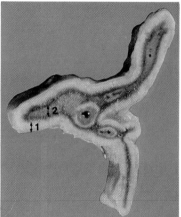

Cross-section
1. cortex　2. medulla

Thymus gland
Though its function has not been determined, it is believed to accelerate the growth of bones and to inhibit that of the sexual glands. Recently shown to have an important role in immunology.

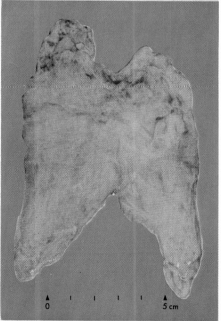

Thymus (adult)
Normally the thymus undergoes complete involution and is turned into fat.

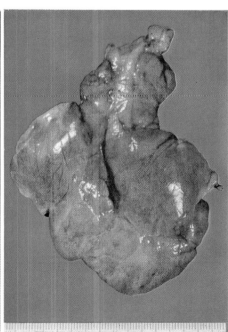

Thymus (child)
A child's thymus consists almost entirely of parenchyma and is large in relation to the body.

As the function of the thymus is not yet known, it has been classified into the endocrine organ. However, it has lately been known to have an important immunological role, that is to say, when the organ is removed in the early stage of development the lymphocytes can not form sufficient antibody. For this reason, the thymus is recently widely regarded as lymphatic tissue.

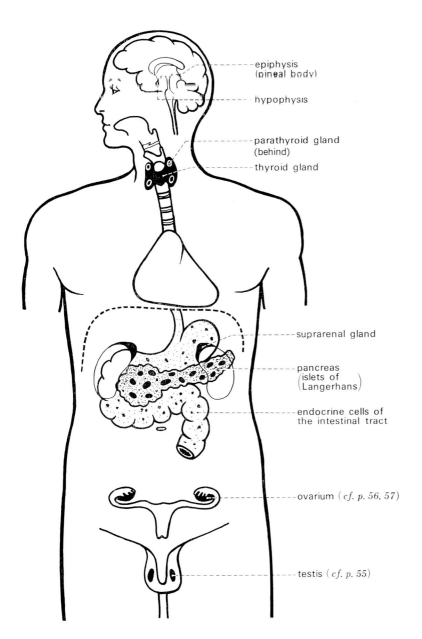

- epiphysis (pineal body)
- hypophysis
- parathyroid gland (behind)
- thyroid gland
- suprarenal gland
- pancreas (islets of Langerhans)
- endocrine cells of the intestinal tract
- ovarium (*cf. p. 56, 57*)
- testis (*cf. p. 55*)

(Superior view, natural size)

Epiphysis (pineal body)
Inhibits manifestation of sex functions.

Hypophysis
(Superior view, natural size)

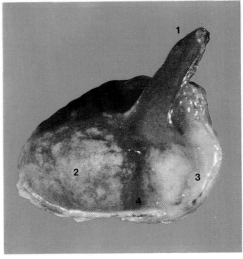

Midsagittal section
1. stalk **2.** anterior lobe **3.** posterior lobe
4. intermediate lobe

Hypophysis

Anterior lobe:
    Growth hormone
    Thyroid stimulating hormone (TSH)
    Corticotropic hormone (ACTH)
Prolactin: stimulates the secretion of milk

Posterior lobe (including the middle lobe):
    Anti-diuretic hormone (ADH)
    Oxytocin contracts the uterus

In contrast to exocrine glands, such as the salivary or intestinal glands that secrete through tubules or ducts, the endocrine glands produce hormones that are absorbed directly into capillaries through which the hormones are distributed throughout the body. Although the amount of secretion is extremely small, chemicals produced by the endocrine system play an essential role in facilitating the metabolic function of the body.

THE MAJOR ARTERIES

1. ant. cerebral artery
2. vertebral a.
3. internal thoracic a.
4. subclavian a.
5. axillary a.
6. aortic arch
7. pulmonary vein
8. intercostal a.
9. superior mesenteric a.
10. lumbar a.
11. common iliac a.
12. internal iliac a.
13. external iliac a.
14. anterior tibial a.
15. posterior tibial a.
16. middle cerebral a.
17. common carotid a.
18. brachiocephalic trunk
19. humeral circumflex a.
20. deep brachial a.
21. brachial a.
22. descending aorta
23. common hepatic a.
24. splenic a.
25. renal a.
26. ulnar a.
27. radial a.
28. inferior mesenteric a.
29. obturator a.
30. internal pudendal a.
31. deep femoral a.
32. femoral a.
33. popliteal a.
34. lateral malleolal a.
   (peroneal a.)
35. lateral plantar a.

HEART

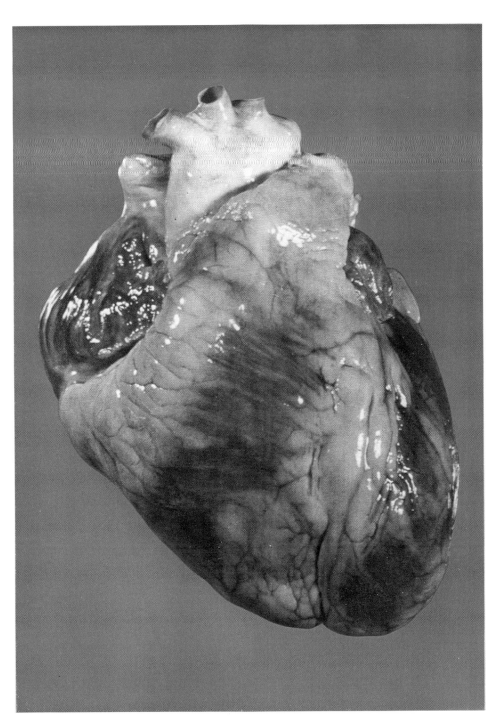

Longitudinally the heart is positioned aslant, its apex directed anteriorly, inferiorly and to the left. In addition, its axis is twisted to the left, so that the anterior view is largely occupied by the right ventricle and only part of the left ventricle and atrium are visible.

The heart is about the size of a closed fist. Anterior view (natural size)

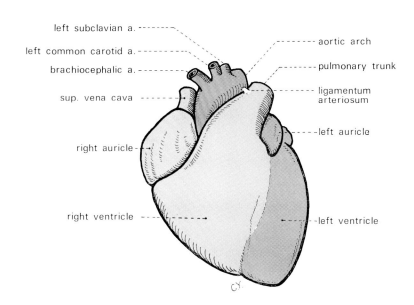

left subclavian a.

left common carotid a.

brachiocephalic a.

sup. vena cava

right auricle

right ventricle

aortic arch

pulmonary trunk

ligamentum arteriosum

left auricle

left ventricle

Relations of Heart to Thorax

A. right atrium
B. left atrium
C. right ventricle
D. left ventricle
1. brachiocephalic trunk (innominate a.)
2. left common carotid artery
3. left subclavian a.
4. aorta
5. ligamentum arteriosum
6. left pulmonary artery
7. right pulmonary artery
8. left pulmonary veins
9. coronary sinus
10. apex
11. coronary sulcus
12. inferior vena cava
13. right pulmonary veins
14. superior vena cava

The shadow of the heart may be observed by means of radiography, which also shows the blood vessels connected with it. Comparison with the photo below reveals that the shadow in the pulmonary hilus is caused by the pulmonary arteries and veins.

Posterior view

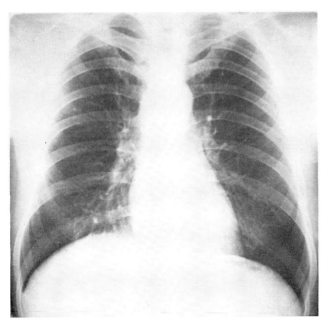

X-ray of the thorax (a — p)

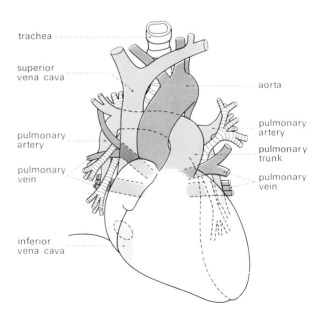

trachea
superior vena cava
pulmonary artery
pulmonary vein
inferior vena cava
aorta
pulmonary artery
pulmonary trunk
pulmonary vein

Anterior view

Nowadays it is possible to replace the heart with an artificial pump, if only for a brief period of time required for an operation of the heart for example. The heart can perform the function of a pump because its four valves are so positioned as to direct the blood flow in one direction only.

The photograph at the right shows a bridge (10) that spans the pulmonary trunk and the aortic arch and serves as a bypass that diverts most of pulmonary circuit blood into the aortic arch before birth.

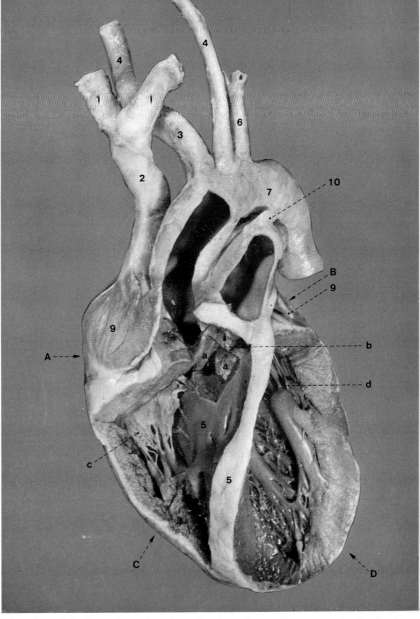

A. right atrium
B. left atrium
C. right ventricle
D. left ventricle
a. cuspis of aortic valve
b. cuspis of pulmonary valve
c. right atrio-ventricular (tricuspid) valve
d. mitral (bicuspid) valve

1. brachiocephalic veins
2. superior vena cava
3. brachiocephalic trune
4. common carotid artery
5. interventricular septum
6. left subclavian artery
7. aorta
8. pulmonary trunk
9. auricle
10. ligamentum arteriosum

Interior of the heart (anterior view). To show the aortic valve and mitral valve the upper part of the interventicular septum is fenestrated.

The direction of blood flow

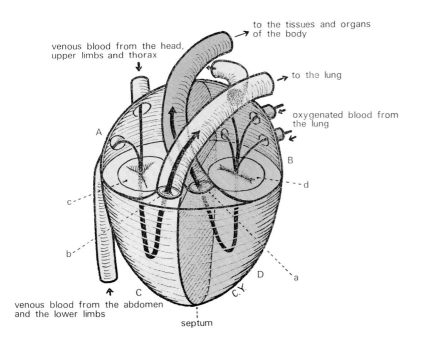

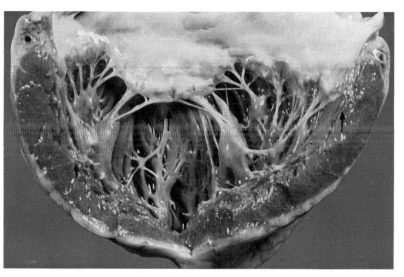

Mitral valve (extended)

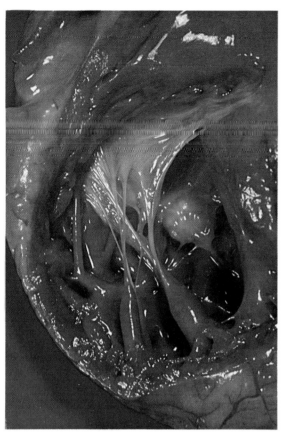

Tricuspid valve (lateral view)

Valves

The mitral valve and the tricuspid valves (atrioventricular valves) have large diameters. To prevent the valve cusps from being forced inside out by a strong pressure caused by the contraction of the ventricle, they are equipped with a number of cords like those of a parachute. Attached to the papillary muscles, they strain with the heart's contraction.

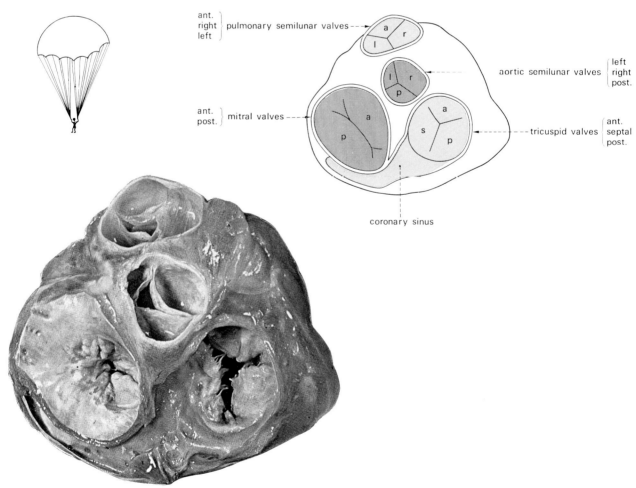

The valves of the heart viewed from base with atria removed, showing orifice and valves (view from above)

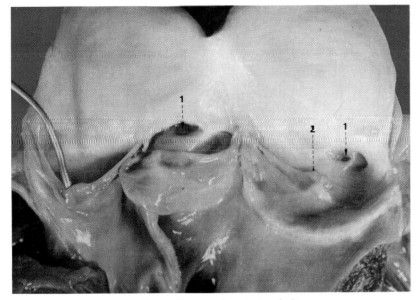

Aortic semilunar valves (extended)
1. opening of coronary aa.   **2.** nodule

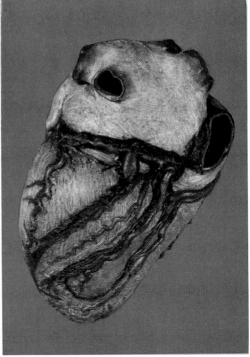

Pulmonary semilunar valve (above: closed) and aortic semilunar valve (below: closed)

Compared to the atrioventricular valves, the aortic semilunar valve and the pulmonary semilunar valve have short diameters and are simply structured with three membranous pouches. The tiny nodes are attached to the edges of the cusps to ensure complete closing of the three cusps.

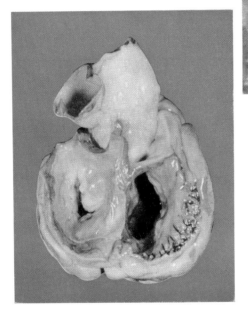

Valvular heart disease:
There are two types of valvular heart disease; one an extreme narrowing of the valves, the other an insufficiency of the valves causing the blood to regurgitate. The photo shows the narrowing of mitral (left) valve.

Blood Supply of the Heart

Coronary arteries and veins:
The blood flowing through the heart is not consumed directly by heart. The myocardium lives on blood distributed by a set of thin blood vessels, the coronary arteries. There are two coronary arteries, each arising from the aorta. When this is closed, fatal diseases such as angina pectoris or myocardial infarction will ensue.

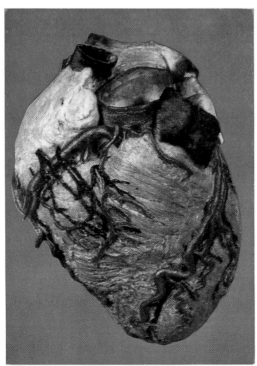

The coronary blood vessels; ventral view (left) and dorsal view (right).

Myocardium and Conducting System

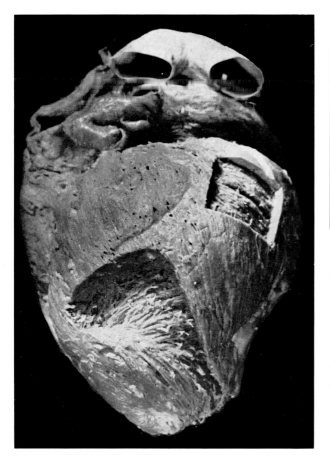

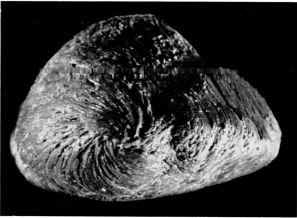

The vortex of the heart: This picture shows the apex of the heart as seen from below. The myocardium is convoluted here like a vortex, hence the name.

The myocardium: The myocardium lies beneath the epicardium, a smooth surface which covers the heart. It consists of two layers in the atrium and three in the ventricle. As the photograph shows, the muscle layers can not be completely distinguished from one another since they merge with each other.

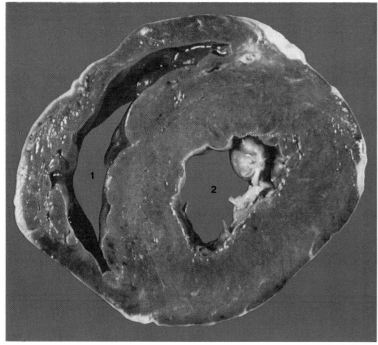

Cross section of ventricles

The wall of the left ventricle is far thicker than that of the right one, because it must withstand the strong pressure required to pump blood throughout the body.

1. right ventricle **2.** left ventricle **3.** right atrium **4.** coronary sinus **5.** superior vena cava **6.** aorta **7.** pulmonary trunk **8.** arterioventricular node **9.** right bundle branch **10.** tricuspid valve **11.** interventricular septum

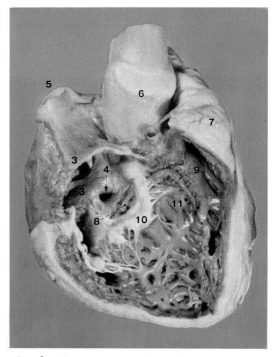

Conduction system of the heart — The interior of the right atrium and of the ventricles, showing the bundle of His: The sinoatrial node in the right atrium generates exciting impulses which spread to the atrioventricular node, then through a bundle of special muscular fibers, the bundle of His (atrioventricular bundle), into the ventricles.

FETAL CIRCULATION

During the fetal period, the uptake of nutrients and of oxygen into the fetus, and the excretion of the metabolites are accomplished via the placenta, and the circulatory system is somewhat different than that of the postnatal life. The blood which has circulated through the fetus is transported to the placenta via umbilical arteries, and then, after the purification, the oxygen rich blood enters the umbilical vein which joins the portal vein in the fetus. However, a large part of the blood returns to the right atrium through the ductus venosus.

A greater part of the blood in the right atrium enters the left one directly via the foramen ovale, then the left ventricle, and finally the aorta. The blood which pours into the right ventricle from the right atrium enters the pulmonary trunk and pours into the aorta via a by-pass named the ductus arteriosus.

1. trachea   2. common carotid artery   3. right brachiocephalic vein   4. superior vena cava   5. *right atrium and foramen ovale*   6. inferior vena cava   7. ductus venosus   8. *umbilical vein*   9. portal vein   10. *ductus arteriosus*   11. aorta   12. pulmonary trunk   13. heart   14. lung   15. stomach   16. small intestine   17. *umbilical cord*   18. *umbilical artery*   19. urachus   20. urinary bladder   21. spleen   22. hepatic a.   23. liver

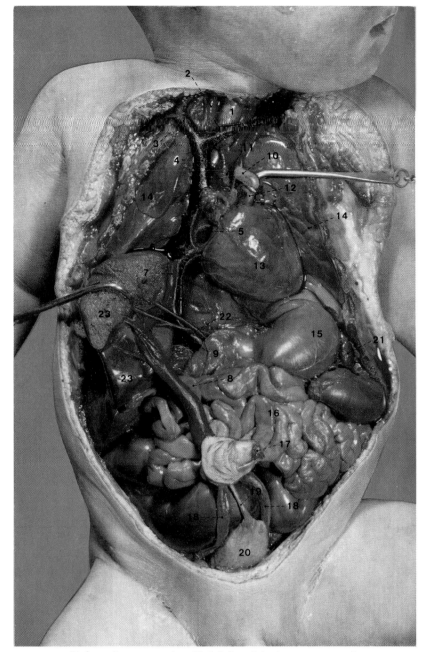

Right atrium opened and left lobe of the liver is resected

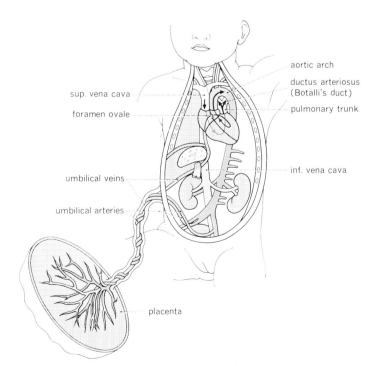

sup. vena cava

foramen ovale

umbilical veins

umbilical arteries

placenta

aortic arch

ductus arteriosus
(Botalli's duct)

pulmonary trunk

inf. vena cava

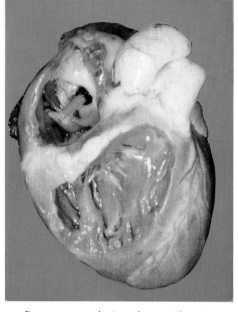

Foramen ovale (newborn infant)
An indicator is inserted into it.

ARTERIES and VEINS

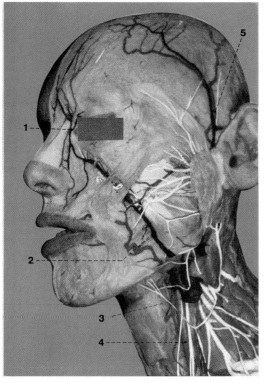

Vessels and nerves of the superficial head and face

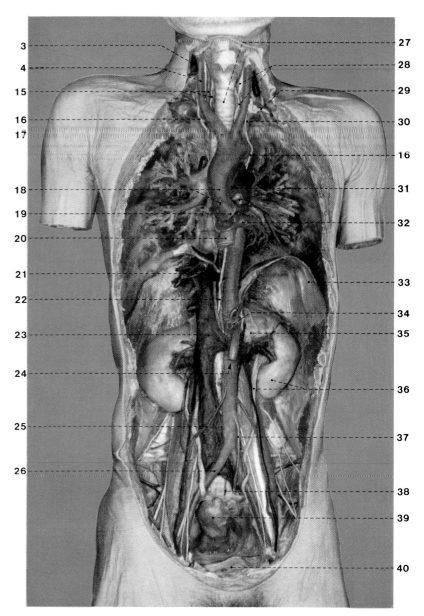

The major vessels of trunk

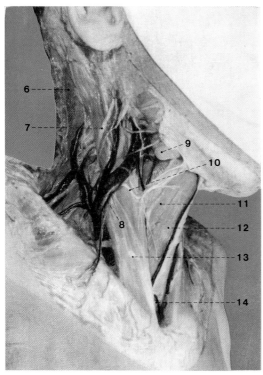

Superficial veins of the neck

1. angular a. and v.
2. facial a. and v.
3. int. jugular v.
4. common carotid a.
5. superficial temporal a. and v.
6. trapezius m.
7. great auricular nerve
8. ext. jugular v.
9. submandibular gland
10. transverse n. of neck
11. omohyoid muscle
12. sternohyoid m.
13. sternomastoid m.
14. ant. jugular v.
15. vertebral a. and recurrent n.
16. vagus n.
17. brachiocephalic a.
18. ascending aorta and right coronary a.
19. aortic valve
20. esophagus
21. hepatic v.
22. thoracic duct
23. inf. vena cava
24. sup. mesenteric a.
25. testicular a.
26. common iliac a.
27. trachea
28. recurrent n. and superior cervical ganglion of sympathetic trunk
29. jugular and subclavian lymphatic trunk
30. subclavian a.
31. pulmonary trunk and valve
32. pulmonary v.
33. diaphragm
34. celiac a. and ganglion
35. suprarenal gland
36. kidney and ureter
37. inf. mesenteric a.
38. middle sacral a.
39. rectum
40. urinary bladder

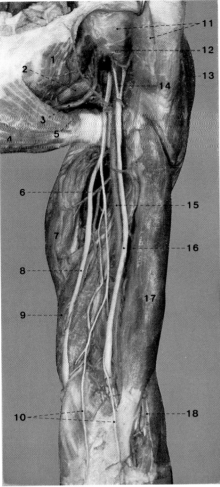

Axilla and arm (left)
(anterior view)

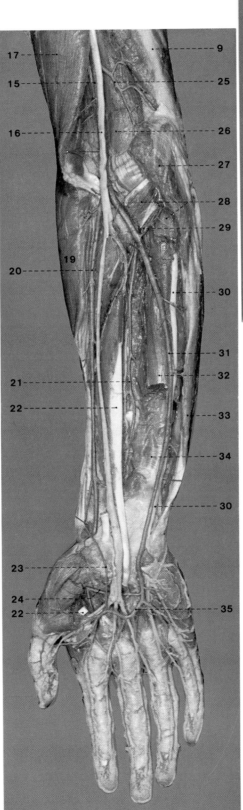

Arteries of the right forearm and hand
(anterior view, deep dissection)

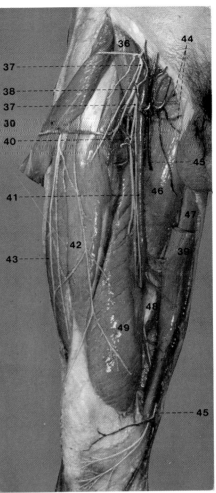

Vessels of the right thigh

Upper limbs

1. serratus anterior m.
2. teres minor m.
3. thoracodorsal a.
4. latissimus dorsi m.
5. scapular circumflex a.
6. profunda brachii a.
7. triceps m. (long)
8. ulnar n.
9. triceps m. (medial)
10. med. antebrachial cutaneous n.
11. pectoralis minor m.
12. brachial v.
13. deltoid m.
14. brachial plexus
15. brachial a.
16. median n.
17. biceps m. (long)
18. lat. antebrachial cutaneous n.

Forearm

19. brachioradialis m.
20. radial a.
21. volar interosseous a.
22. flexor pollicis longus m.
23. superficial palmar branch
24. deep palmar arch
25. inf. ulnar collateral a.
26. brachialis m.
27. flexor m. (common origin)
28. pronator teres m.
29. ulnar recurrent a.
30. ulnar n.
31. ulnar a.
32. flex. digitor. profundus m.
33. flex. carpi ulnaris m.
34. pronator quadratus m.
35. superficial palmar arch

Leg

36. iliopsoas m.
37. femoral a.
38. sup. epigastric a. and circumflex. iliac a.
39. sartorius
40. ant. femoral cutaneous n.
41. femoral a.
42. rectus femoris m.
43. vastus lateralis m.
44. external pudendal a.
45. great saphenous v.
46. adductor longus m.
47. gracilis m.
48. adductor magnus m.
49. vastus medialis m.

Compared with arteries, veins have thin walls and smaller internal pressure, which is liable to cause blood to flow backwards. To prevent regurgitation most veins have valves located along their course. Venous valves are absent in the head but are abundant in the extremity.

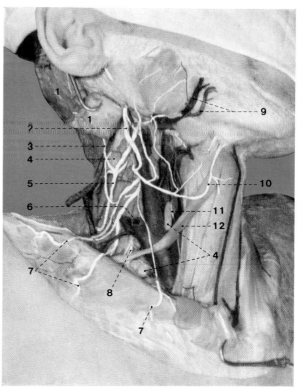

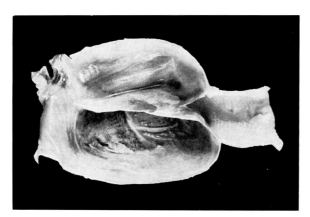

A bicuspid valve in a vein

Internal jugular vein (center)

1. sternocleidomastoid m.　**2.** great auricular n.　**3.** lesser occipital n.　**4.** lymph node　**5.** accessory n.　**6.** external jugular vein　**7.** supraclavicular n.　**8.** cervical n.　**9.** facial a. and v.　**10.** transverse n.　**11.** common carotid a. and descending branch of hypoglossal n.　**12.** omohyoid m.

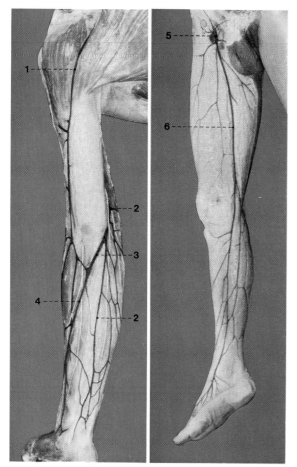

The superficial veins of the upper limb (left) and the lower limb (right)

Most veins run parallel with arteries, but subcutaneous veins run their own independent course. They interwine to form networks so that the interruption of blood circulation does not occur when pressure is applied partially.

1. cephalic v.　**2.** basilic v.　**3.** vena mediana cubiti **4.** median antebrachial v.　**5.** femoral a. and v.　**6.** great saphenous v.

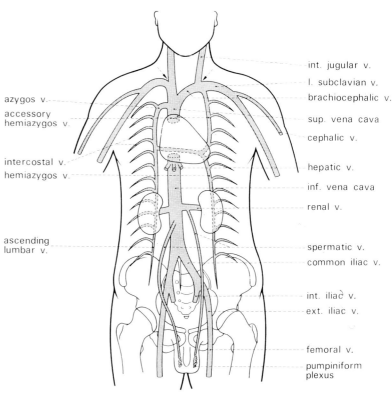

The main veins of the body
(Arrows: right and left angulus venosus)

azygos v.
accessory hemiazygos v.
intercostal v.
hemiazygos v.
ascending lumbar v.

int. jugular v.
l. subclavian v.
brachiocephalic v.
sup. vena cava
cephalic v.
hepatic v.
inf. vena cava
renal v.
spermatic v.
common iliac v.
int. iliac v.
ext. iliac v.
femoral v.
pumpiniform plexus

LYMPHATIC VESSELS and LYMPH NODES

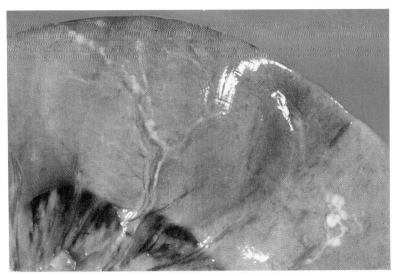

Lymphatic vessels of small intestine
The lymph in the lymph vessel of the small intestine contains a lot of fat droplets and looks white.

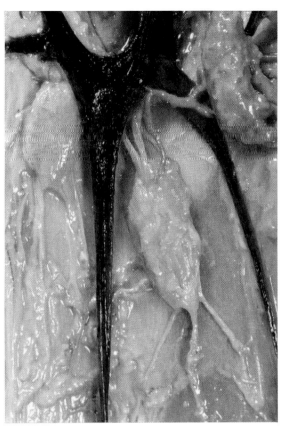

Inguinal lymph nodes

Lymph vessels collect lymphatic fluid from the body tissues and ultimately empty into veins. The lymph nodes along the way do not capture harmful bacteria alone but rather produce antibodies. Structurally, lymph vessels closely resemble veins but they have more valves. This gives them the appearance of a string of beads.

SPLEEN

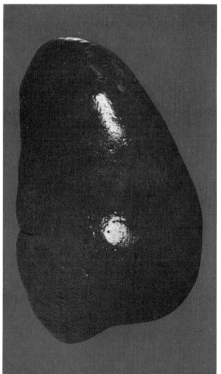

Diaphragmatic surface

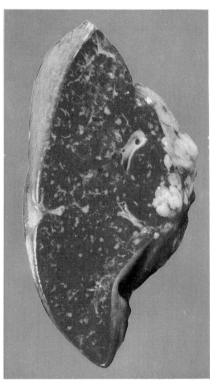

Cross-section
The white dots in figure are the white pulp.

The spleen is an organ located to the left rear of the stomach. Its size is largely dependent on the amount of blood, but the average length is about 10 cm. It belongs to the lymphatic system and produces lymphocytes. It also destroys old red cells, which in turn serve as material for bile or new red cells. Man can live when the spleen is removed in an operation.

On the other hand it serves as a blood depository. One sometimes feels pain in the left upper abdomen when running immediately after eating. This pain results from a sudden contraction of the spleen. During digestion, blood converges in the digestive organs. But running necessitates that a large supply of blood be pumped to the muscles at the same time. Consequently, the spleen contracts to give up its own blood supply.

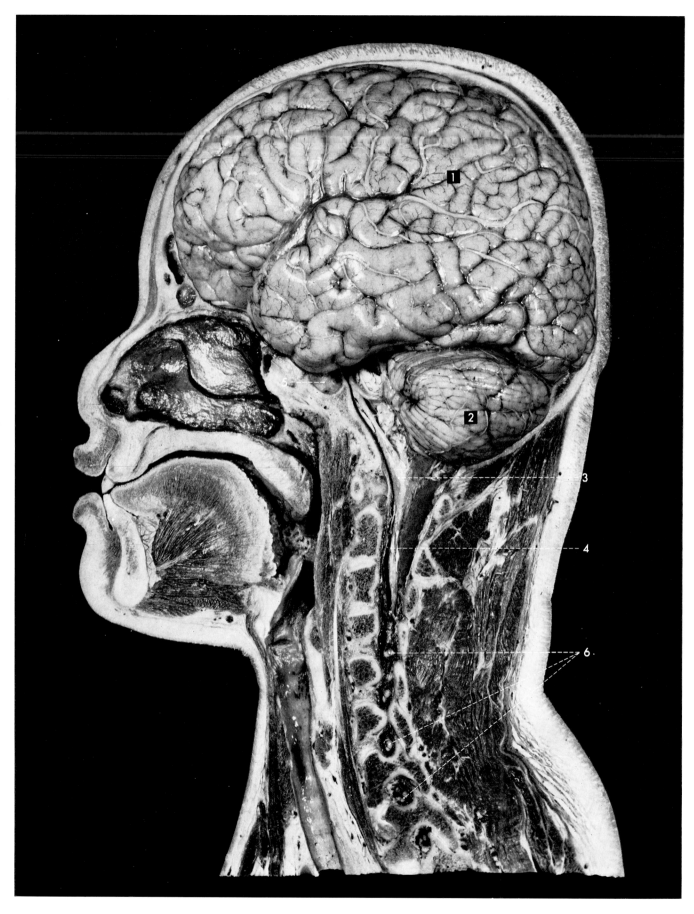

CENTRAL NERVOUS SYSTEM

The midbrain is hidden from view

1. cerebrum
2. cerebellum
3. medulla oblongata
4. spinal cord
5. hypophysis
6. spinal nerves

Brain

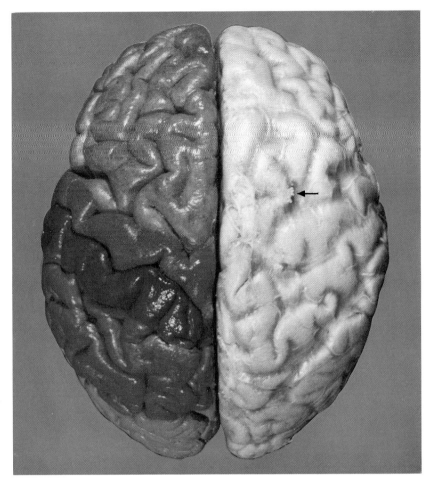

Left hemisphere is colored (cf. p. 82).
Red: Frontal lobe
Purple: Parietal lobe
Green: Occipital lobe
Dark red: Precentral gyrus
Dark blue: Postcentral gyrus
Arrow: Arachnoid granulation

Cerebral hemisphere, viewed from above. Right hemisphere is covered with arachnoid.

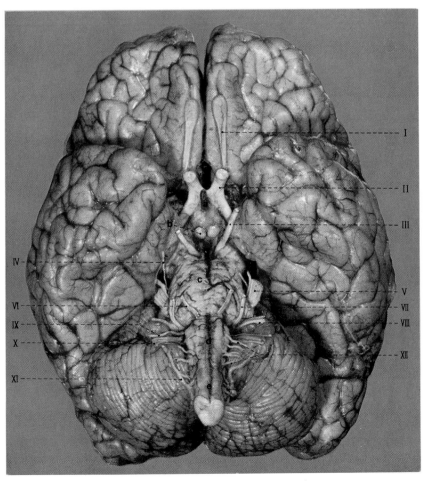

I. olfactory tract
II. optic nerve
III. oculomotor n.
IV. trochlear n.
V. trigeminal n.
VI. abducent n.
VII. facial n.
VIII. statoacoustic n.
IX. glossopharyngeal n.
X. vagus n.
XI. accessory n.
XII. hypoglossal n.

a. infundibulum
b. mammillary body
c. pons
d. medulla oblongata
e. pyramidal decussation

Base of the brain, showing position of cranial nerves.

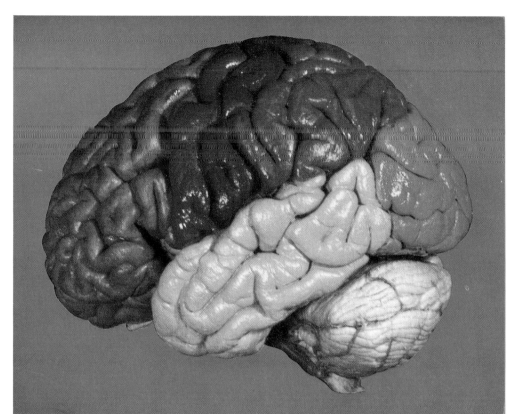

Red: Frontal lobe
Purple: Parietal lobe
Green: Occipital lobe
Yellow: Temporal lobe

Lateral aspect of left cerebral hemisphere

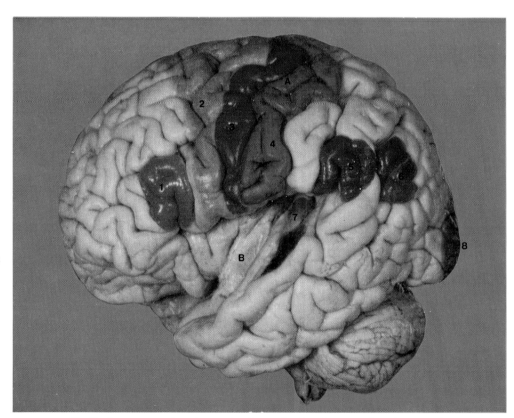

A. central sulcus
B. Insula (lateral sulcus is opened)

1. motor-speech area
2. pre-motor area
3. somato-motor area
4. somato-sensory area
5. speech understanding center
6. reading center
7. acoustic area (red: high tone, blue: low tones)
8. visual-sensory centers

Cortical sensory and motor center. Lateral sulcus is opened to show insula

Locations of cerebral cortex functions

The cortex of the cerebral hemisphere has definite functional areas. The most interesting observation will be made on both sides of the central sulcus that runs longitudinally across the approximate center of the cerebral hemisphere. The frontal part of the sulcus is a center of somato-motor functions, whereas the posterior part controls somato-sensory functions.

Like a man standing on his head, the inferior part governs the head and neck and the superior part the legs.

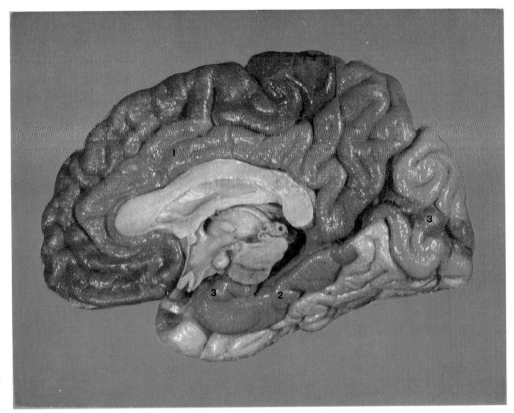

Orange (limbic zone):
1. cingulate gyrus
2. hippocampal gyrus
3. uncus (smell?)
Dark green: Visual area

Medial aspect of right hemisphere

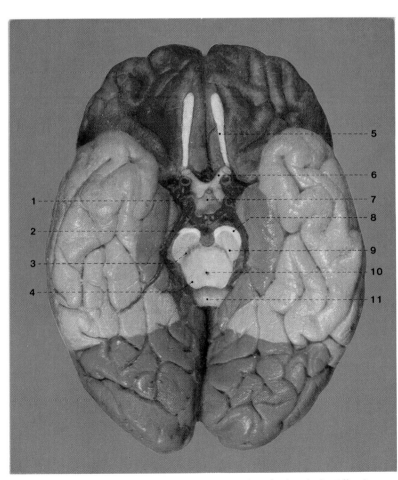

1. circle of Willis
2. posterior cerebral artery
3. substantia nigra
4. superior colliculus
5. olfactory tract
6. optic nerve
7. infundibulum of hypophysis
8. oculomotor nerve
9. cerebral peduncle
10. aqueduct of Sylvius
11. splenium of corpus callosum

Base of brain. Brain stem has been removed at the level of midbrain.

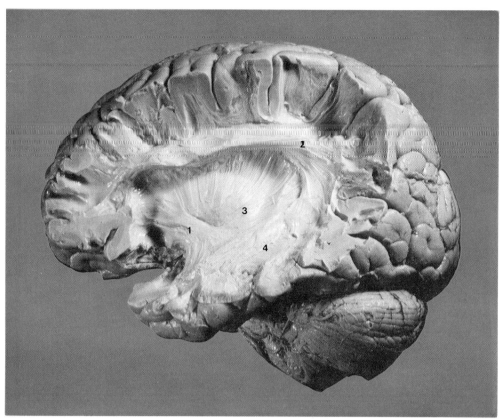

1. uncinate bundle
2. superior longitudinal bundle
3. external capsule
4. inferior longitudinal bundle

White substance consists of many nerve fibers. Long association fibers connect distant parts of cortex.

Principal association bundles disseted from lateral view.

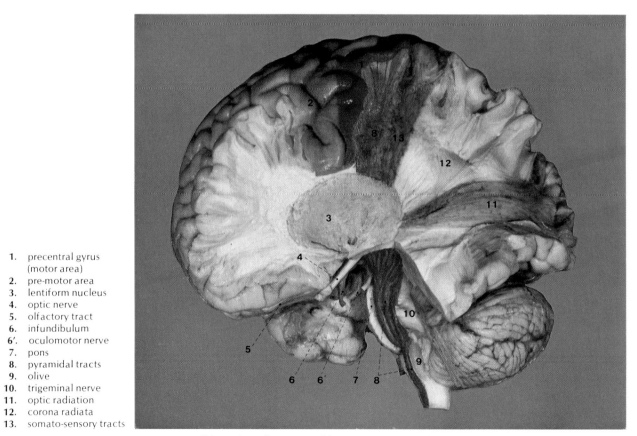

1. precentral gyrus (motor area)
2. pre-motor area
3. lentiform nucleus
4. optic nerve
5. olfactory tract
6. infundibulum
6'. oculomotor nerve
7. pons
8. pyramidal tracts
9. olive
10. trigeminal nerve
11. optic radiation
12. corona radiata
13. somato-sensory tracts

Dissection of cortex and brain stem. Pyramidal system and optic system.

1. caudate nucleus
2. lentiform nucleus
3. corpus callosum (splenium)
4. anterior cerebral artery
5. amygdala
6. a portion of left medial orbital gyrus
7. olfactory tract
8. optic nerve
9. internal carotid a. and infundibulum
10. oculomotor nerve
11. basilar artery
12. trigeminal nerve
13. abducent n.
14. facial n.
15. vestibulocochlear n.
16. hypoglosal n.
17. olive
18. pyramidal tract
19. internal capsule
20. anterior commissure
21. amygdaloid body
22. cerebral peduncle
23. trochlear n.
24. inferior colliculus
25. posterior cerebral artery
26. superior cerebellar peduncle
27. inferior cerebellar peduncle
28. middle cerebellar peduncle
29. glossopharyngeal n.
30. vagus n.

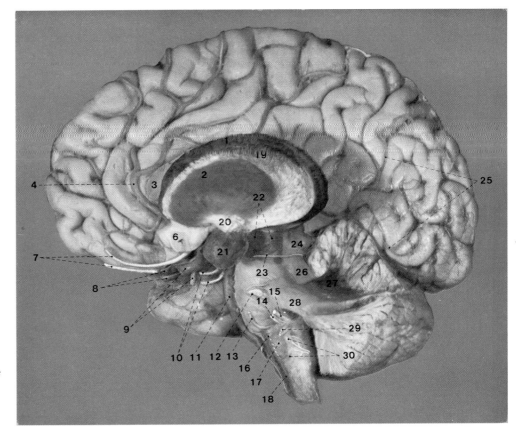

Brain stem (lateral view), Pyramidal tract and cerebellar peduncles

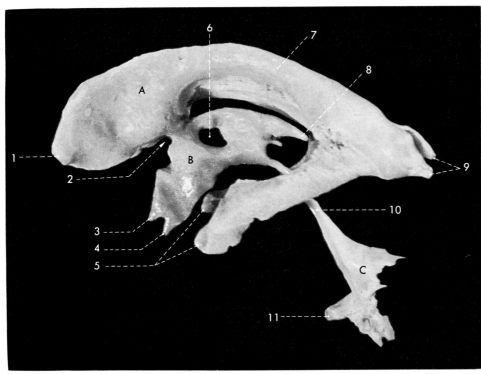

Cast of the ventricular cavities, viewed from the left side.

A. lateral ventricle
B. third ventricle
C. fourth ventricle

1. anterior horn
2. interventricular foramen
3. optic recessus
4. infundibulum
5. inferior horn
6. massa intermedia
7. body
8. suprapineal recess
9. posterior horn (right and left)
10. cerebral aqueduct
11. lateral recess

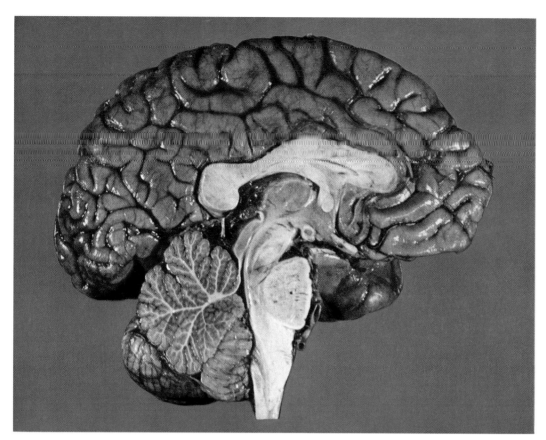

Midsagittal section of the brain. Right cerebral hemisphere (medial aspect)

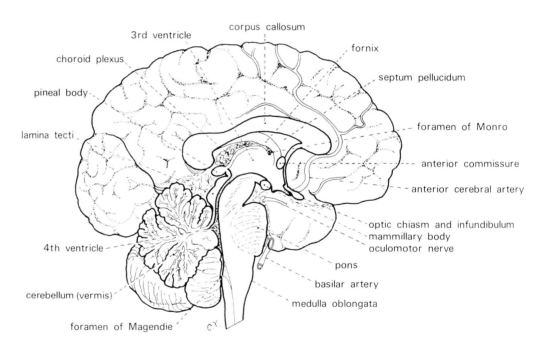

The brainstem is so covered by the cerebral hemisphere that the upper half is externally invisible. It contains the center essential to life preservation. The majority of the cerebral nerves originate here. Due to the under-developed cerebral hemisphere, the brainstem of lower animals is exposed.

The brainstem consists of the following parts.

BRAINSTEM
- interbrain (thalamus, hypothalamus)
- midbrain (tectum, tegmentum, cerebral peduncle)
- pons
- medulla oblongata

In brief, the brainstem is that which remains after the cerebral hemisphere and cerebellum are removed.
Note: The tegmentum lies between the tectum and cerebral peduncle and is scarcely visible from the surface.

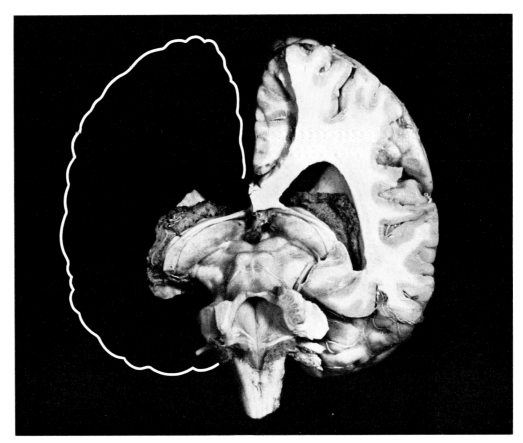

Brainstem (dorsal view). Left cerebral hemisphere, cerebellum and dorsal half of the right hemisphere are removed, and rhomboid fossa is shown.

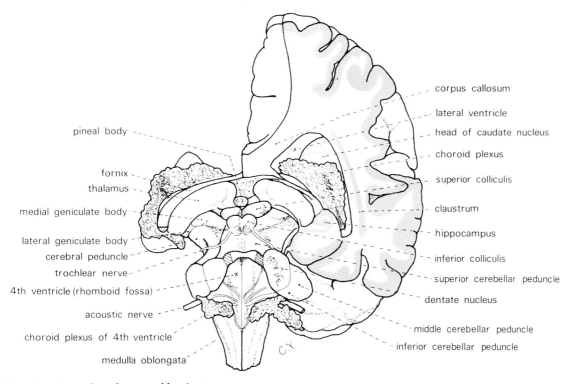

pineal body

fornix
thalamus
medial geniculate body

lateral geniculate body
cerebral peduncle
trochlear nerve
4th ventricle (rhomboid fossa)
acoustic nerve
choroid plexus of 4th ventricle
medulla oblongata

corpus callosum
lateral ventricle
head of caudate nucleus
choroid plexus
superior colliculis
claustrum
hippocampus
inferior colliculis
superior cerebellar peduncle
dentate nucleus
middle cerebellar peduncle
inferior cerebellar peduncle

The function of each part of brainstem

The thalamus is concerned with perception. Every perceptive impulse reaches the cerebral cortex through the thalamus. Its function is also connected with emotion and feeling.

The hypothalamus is the control center for temperature, water, sleep and digestion. The pituitary body is attached to it.

The midbrain is the center which influences the posture and extrapyramidal movements, autonomic reflexes and regulates movement of the eyeballs, and adjusts pupils and posture, etc.

The pons consists of scattered cell groups (pontic nuclei) and transverse fibers which arise from the nuclei and pass into the cerebellum (commissure fibers of the cerebellum).

The medulla oblongata is a vital center that controls respiration, heartbeat, biting, swallowing, vomiting, speech and secretion of saliva and tears.

Internal Features of the Brain (frontal section)

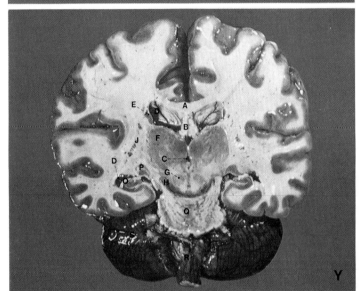

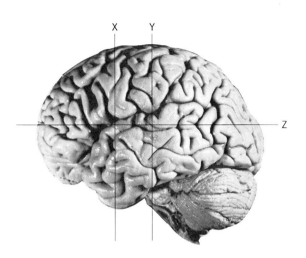

Frontal section

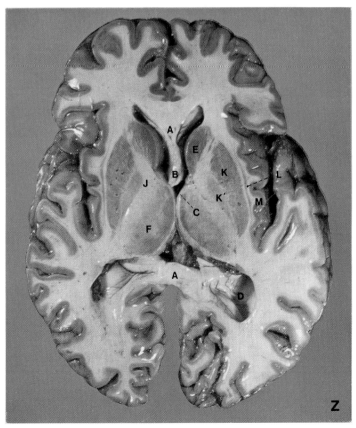

Horizontal section

The brain consists of nerve cells and nerve fibers. The former have a tendency to gather at the surface of the brain. Groups of nerve cells appear gray, hence the name "gray matter" or cortex. As numerous nerve cells are crowded into the limited space, the surface of the brain is wrinkled to increase the surface area. Those cells that do not form part of the surface are found in an independent group of nerve cells in the center, known as the nucleus. The remaining whitish part is called either medulla or white substance and consists of nerve fibers. The cerebral cortex of an adult is said to have nearly 16,400,000,000 nerve cells.

A. corpus callosum
B. fornix
C. third ventricle
D. lateral ventricle
E. caudate nucleus
F. thalamus
G. red nucleus
H. substantia nigra
I. optic tract
J. internal capsule
K. putamen
K'. globus pallidus } lentiform nucleus

L. claustrum
M. insula
N. amygdaloid body
O. hippocampus
P. lateral geniculate body
Q. pons
R. medulla oblongata
S. cerebellum

Spinal Cord

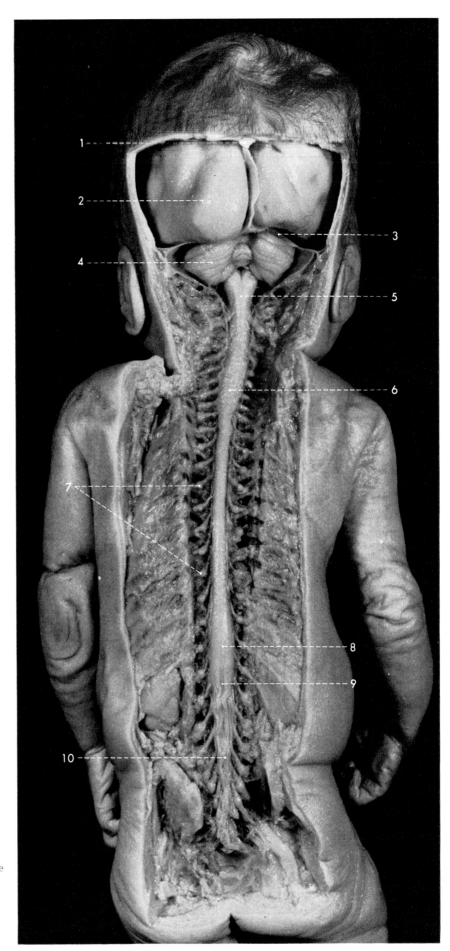

1. falx cerebri
2. cerebral hemisphere
3. tentorium cerebelli
4. cerebellar hemisphere
5. medulla oblongata
6. cervical enlargement
7. spinal ganglions
8. lumbar enlargement
9. conus medullaris
10. cauda equina

The brain and spinal cord (matured fetus)
The spinal cord is exposed from behind. Thirty-one pairs of spinal nerves emerge from the spinal cord. The posterior root presents a spinal ganglion. Cervical enlargement and lumbar enlargement are expanded because the brachial and leg nerves originate from them respectively. The spinal cord terminates just below the lumbar enlargement. Beyond this point the spinal nerves form a bundle to become cauda equina.
   Also note that embryo's cerebrum has fewer wrinkles.

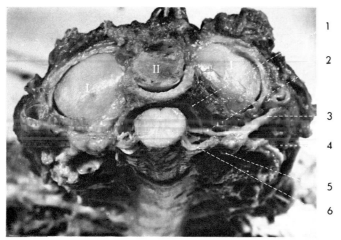

Superoposterior view

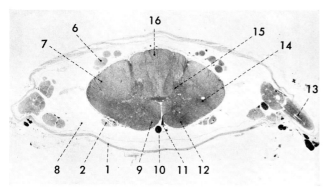

Lateral view

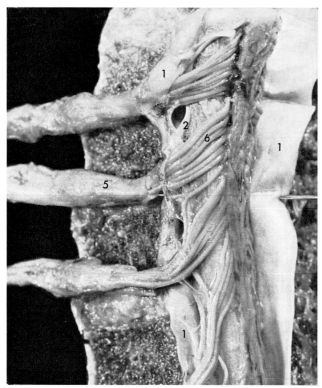

Cross-section for photomicrograph (c.v.)

Spinal cord and nerves

I. superior articular surface **II.** dentoid process (2nd cervical vertebrae)

1. dura mater **2.** anterior root **3.** anterior ramus **4.** posterior ramus **5.** spinal ganglion **6.** posterior root **7.** lateral funiculus **8.** subarachnoid space **9.** anterior funiculus **10.** anterior spinal artery **11.** anterior median fissure **12.** anterior column **13.** spinal nerve **14.** lateral column **15.** posterior column **16.** posterior funiculus

The spinal cord is encased in the bony spinal canal and is protected by thick dura mater. The anterior root consists of motor nerve fibers and the posterior root of sensory nerve fibers, both of which combine to become spinal nerves. They are divided into frontal ramus and posterior ramus.

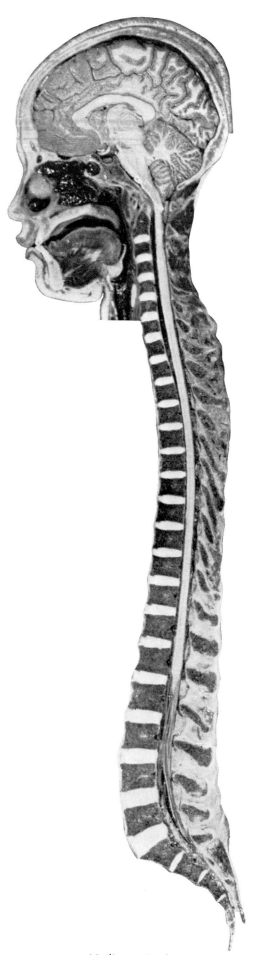

Median sagittal section

PERIPHERAL NERVES

Every organ above the neck is innervated by brain nerves that emerge out directly from the brain. There are twelve pairs of these. The nerves below the neck energe out from the spinal cord, i. e. spinal nerves, and there are thirty-one pairs of these. Only the representative nerves will be mentioned here.

The neck being the boundary, both brain nerves and spinal nerves co-exist.

Facial nerve
The facial nerve innervates the muscles of facial expression and scalp. It gives rise to a number of branches radially through the parotid gland. In palsy, the affected side is flaccid, expressionless, the naso-labial furrow is obliterated, the corner of the mouth droops, the eye can only be partly closed and tears flow over the cheek (Bell's palsy).

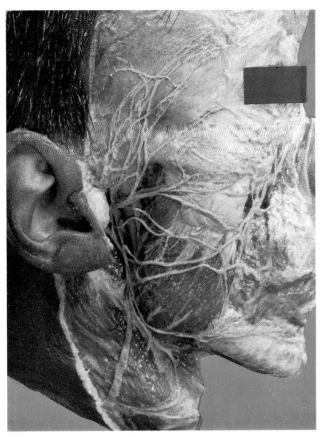

Facial nerve

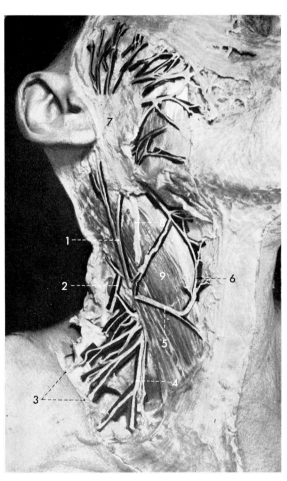

Nerves of the neck and face

1. great auricular n. **2.** post. supraclavicular n. **3.** middle supraclavicular n. **4.** ant. supraclavicular n. **5.** transverse cervical n. **6.** cervical branchi of facial n. **7.** parotid gl. **8.** ext. jugular v. **9.** sternocleidomastoid m. **10.** axillary n. **11.** musculocutaneous n. **12.** ulnar n. **13.** radial n. **14** median n. **15.** med. brachial cutaneous n. **16.** axillary a. and v. **L:** lateral cord of brachial plexus **P:** posterior c. of brachial plexus **M:** medial c. of brachial plexus

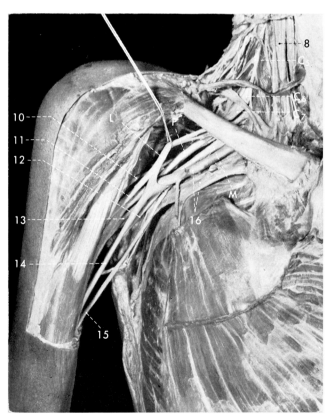

Brachial plexus
Nerves that innervate the arms do not lead directly from the spinal cord, but first form a network of nerves known as the brachial plexus, from which they branch off ($C_5 — Th_1$).

Autonomic Nervous System

Sympathetic trunk and vagus

Yellow: sympathetic nerves
Green: parasympathetic (vagus) nerves

1. superior cervical ganglion
2. middle cervical ganglion
3. subclavian artery
4. stellate ganglion and ansa subclavia
5. rami communicantes
6. greater splanchnic nerve
7. lesser splanchnic n.
8. sympathetic trunk
9. splanchnic nerve
   (enters the celiac ganglion)
10. sucostal nerve (Th12)
11. common carotid artery
12. trachea
13. brachial plexus
14. vagus nerve
15. esophagus
16. recurrent nerve
17. azygos vein
18. aortic hiatus of diaphragm
19. iliohypogastric n.
20. ilioinguinal n.
21. femoral n.
22. lateral cutaneous nerve of thigh
23. genitofemoral n.
24. obturator n.
25. femoral artery
26. intercostal nerve

Intercostal nerves

Nerves originating in the spinal cord (spinal nerves) are divided into anterior ramus and posterior ramus. The latter supply the adjacent back muscles or skin overlying them, but the former form a nerve plexus, from which the nerves arise.

The only exception is the group of thoracic nerves, which run directly to the side and the anterior of the body. Called intercostal nerves, they innervate not only the chest but also the greater part of the abdominal wall.

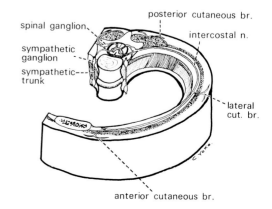

spinal ganglion
sympathetic ganglion
sympathetic trunk
posterior cutaneous br.
intercostal n.
lateral cut. br.
anterior cutaneous br.

Nerves of Extremities

Upper limb

1. teres minor
2. deltoid
3. superficial epigastric vessels and superficial ext. pudendal vessels
4. profunda brachii a. (radial and middle branch)
5. radial nerve
6. triceps (lateral head)
7. scapular circumflex
8. teres major
9. triceps (medial head)
10. latissimus dorsi
11. median n.
12. ulnar n.
13. olecranon

Lower limb

14. gluteus medius
15. gluteus minimus
16. greater trochanter
17. quadratus femoris
18. gluteus maximus
19. adductor minimus
20. adductor magnus
21. sciatic n.
22. biceps femoris (short head)
23. biceps femoris (long head)
24. common peroneal n. and lateral sural cutaneous
25. gastrocnemius
26. piriformis
27. gemelli and obturator internus
28. ischial tuberosity
29. semitendinosus
30. gracilis
31. semimembranosus
32. tibial n.
33. medial sural cutaneous n.
34. superficial iliac circum-flex artery and vein
35. lateral femoral cutan-eous n.
36. femoral a. and v.
37. anterior cutaneous branches of femoral n.
38. superficial epigastric a. and v.
39. femoral n.
40. superficial epigastric vessels and superficial ext. pudendal vessels
41. great saphenous v.
42. saphenous n.
43. popliteus

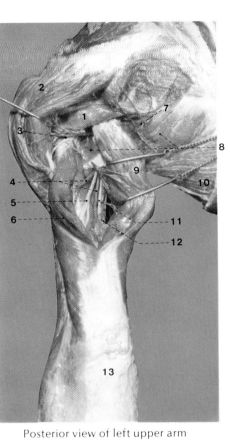

Posterior view of left upper arm

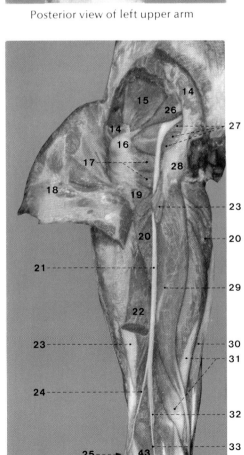

Posterior view of the left gluteal and femoral regions

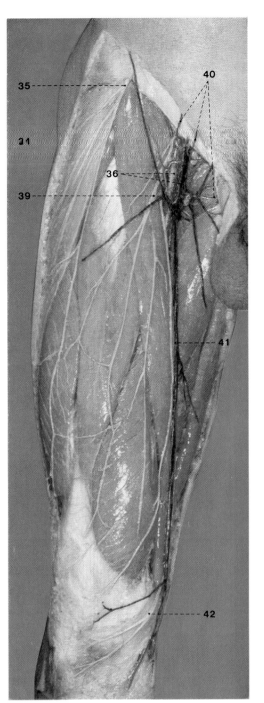

Cutaneous nerves and superficial vessels of right thigh

The sciatic nerve is the longest of the peripheral nerves. It arises from the lumbar plexus. It is as thick as the little finger at its root and measures as long as 1 m. Consequently, it is quite prone to neuralgia. It also innervates all the muscles on the posterior side of the lower limb.

EAR

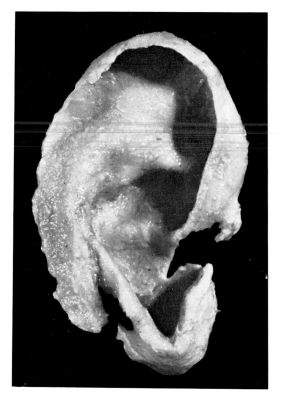

The cartilage of the auricle (pinna)

The ear is the organ of hearing and balance. The former function is controlled by the eardrum, ossicles which transmit vibrations of the eardrum to the inner ear, and the cochlea that perceives sounds in the inner ear. Balance is controlled by semicircular canals which contain fluid. There are physical devices that perceive the movement of the fluid brought on by the movement of the body, and enable one to tell the position of his head or his motion.

The auricle contains a highly elastic cartilage which maintains its shape. In spite of the supposed significance of the intricately irregular shape, the curvature of the auricle seems to have little acoustic significance.

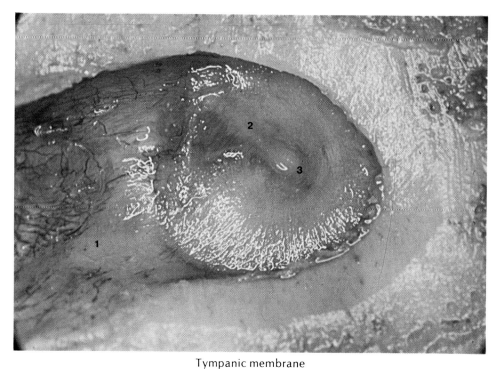

Tympanic membrane
1. external acoustic meatus   **2.** handle of malleus   **3.** umbo

The membrane of the tympanum is of an irregular oval shape. It is 9.4 mm in length but only 0.1 mm thick. Because it is translucent, the malleus attached to it from the inside can be seen through it. The center is called the navel.

External Ear and Middle Ear

Ear consists of three parts: the external ear (outside of eardrum), middle ear (tympanic cavity), and internal ear (labyrinth).

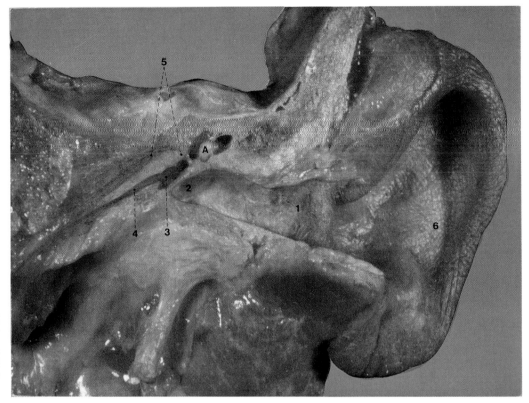

The external ear and the middle ear (anterior view)

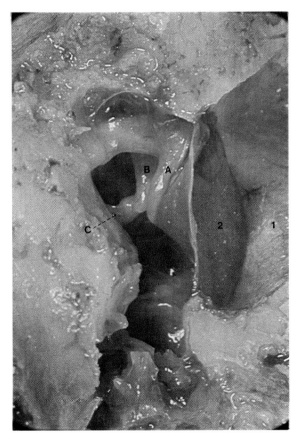

Tympanic membrane and chain ossicles

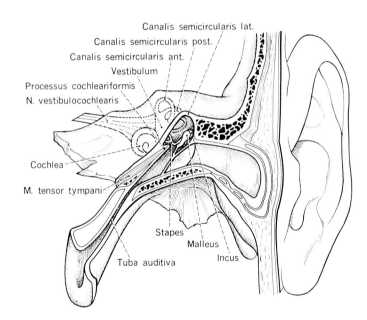

Canalis semicircularis lat.
Canalis semicircularis post.
Canalis semicircularis ant.
Vestibulum
Processus cochleariformis
N. vestibulocochlearis
Cochlea
M. tensor tympani
Stapes
Malleus
Incus
Tuba auditiva

A. malleus
B. incus
C. stapes
1. external acoustic meatus
2. tympanic membrane
3. tympanic cavity
4. auditory tube
5. tensor tympani
6. auricle

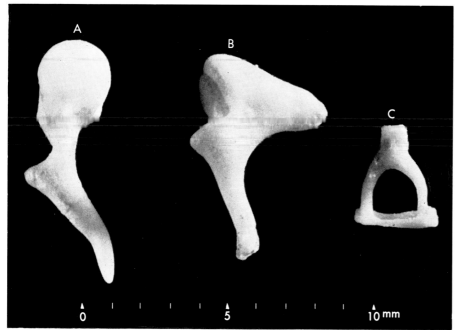

A. malleus
B. incus
C. stapes

Auditory ossicles:
The auditory ossicles consist of three bones. The innermost stapes is attached to the oval window. When it vibrates, the vibration is transmitted to the fluid inside the cochlea. As a result we perceive sounds.

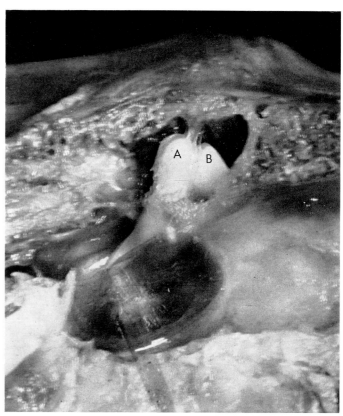

The movement of the ear bones
This picture shows the vibrations of ossicles with the vibrations of eardrum which were caused mechanically by a stick.

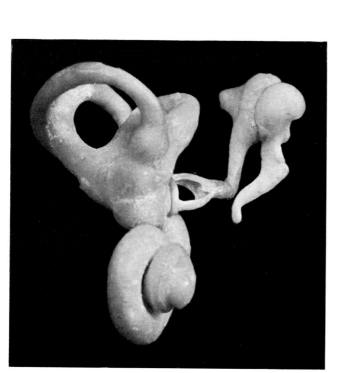

Chain ossicles and labyrinth

Internal Ear or Labyrinth

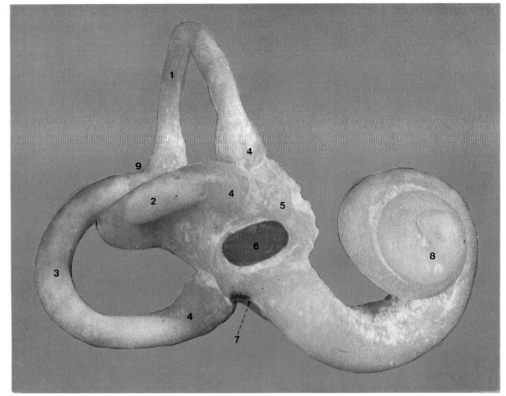

1. superior semicircular canal
2. lateral s.c.
3. posterior s.c.
4. ampulla
5. vestibule
6. oval window (vestibular fenestra)
7. round window (cochlear fenestra)
8. cochlea
9. internal acoustic meatus

A cast of the right internal ear (perilymphatic cavity)

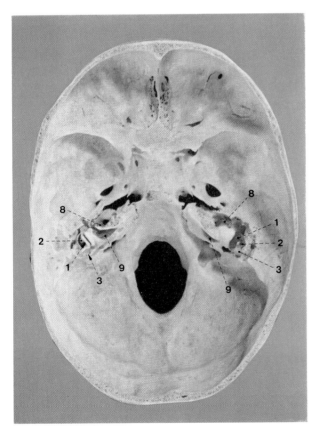

Interior of base of the skull, showing osseous labyrinth
As the labyrinth is embedded within the pyramid of the temporal bone, a portion of the bone must be chipped off to expose it. Left osseous labyrinth is exposed the interior.

The internal ear consists of the semicircular canals and cochlea which are embedded in the petrous portion of the temporal bone. The former is concerned with the function of maintaining equilibrium and the latter with that of analysis of sound. The base of the stapes which fits the oval window transfers the vibration of the tympanum to the lymph in the inner ear. The vibration of the lymph is caught in the spiral organ in the cochlea as a sound.

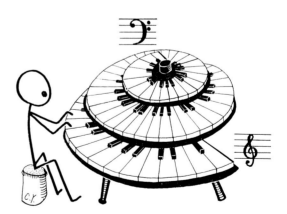

The tip of the cochlea is sensitive to low-pitched sounds, whereas its base is sensitive to high-pitched sounds.

EYE

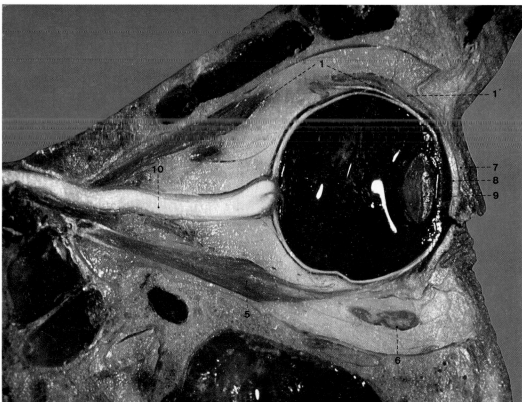

Midsagittal section

1. superior rectus muscle
1'. levator palpebrae superior m.
2. lateral rectus m.
3. superior oblique m.
3'. trochlea
4. medial rectus m.
5. inferior rectus m.
6. inferior oblique m.
7. eyelid
8. tarsus
9. lens
10. optic nerve

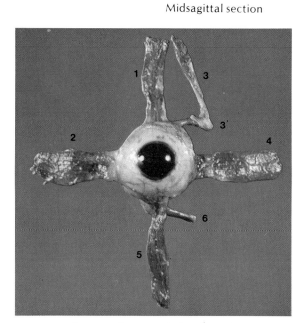

Eye muscles extended (right eye)

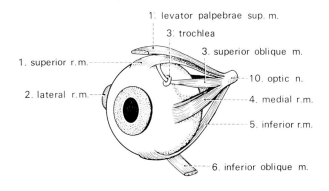

1. levator palpebrae sup. m.
3. trochlea
3. superior oblique m.
1. superior r.m.
10. optic n.
2. lateral r.m.
4. medial r.m.
5. inferior r.m.
6. inferior oblique m.

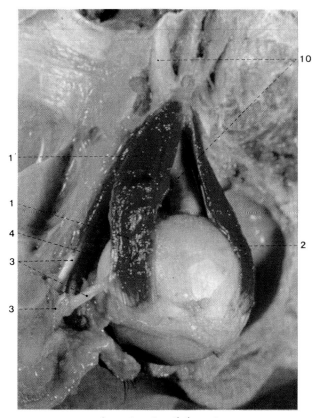

Superior view (left eye)

This picture shows clearly how the superior oblique muscle passes through the trochlea to change direction. The levator palpebrae superioris muscle parallels the rectus bulbi superior muscle. To prevent the upper eyelid from obstructing vision, the latter contracts with the former.

Lens

The lens is suspended from the ciliary body by means of numerous fine fibers. When the ciliary body contracts, these fibers relax and the crystalline lens contracts by its own elasticity to grow thicker. As a result, the light rays passing through the lens are bent to a greater degree and the focal length decreases.

These fibers are microscopic, but in the photograph intertwined fibers can be seen with the naked eye.

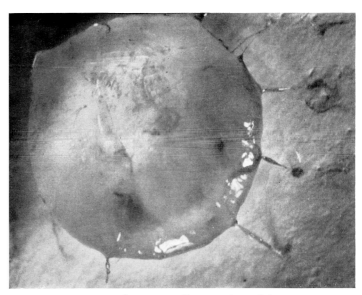

Suspensory ligament (zonula)

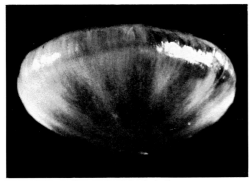

Lens: equatorial view
Above: anterior pole

The lens is nearly 9 mm in diameter. Its thickness is 3.7 mm when focused on a distant object and 4.4 mm. when focused on a near object. The average thickness is 4 mm. The front is slightly less curved.

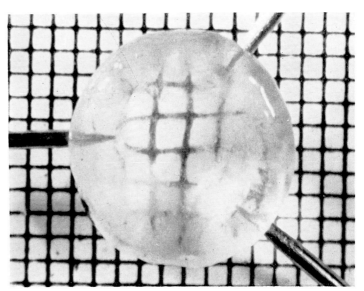

Frontal view of lens

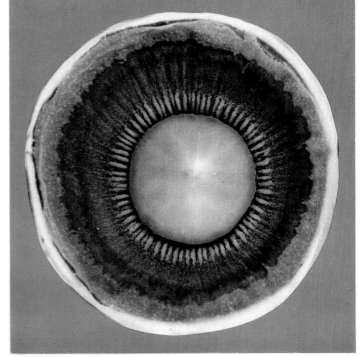

The eyeball is cut along the equator and seen from the inside. The worm-like matter surrounding the lens is the ciliary body, to which the suspensory ligament that suspends the lens adheres. The retina looks dark brown in a cadaver but when alive, it appears bright orange as shown on the next page. Discoloration is said to occur within a few minutes after death.

Ciliary body, Interior of anterior half of bulb

99

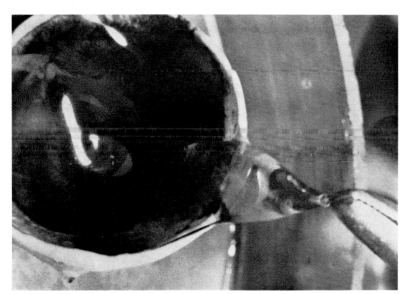

Vitreous Body

Behind the lens, the cavity of the eyeball is filled with a gelatinous transparent material called vitreous body. This substance is so viscous that it can be grasped with forceps. The pupil can be seen beyond.

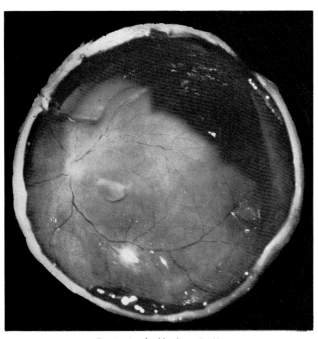

Posterior half of eyeball

Retina

The retina corresponds to a dry plate in photography; at the focus point there is a slight yellowish area (macula lutea) which is the location of sharpest vision. A white circular plate called the papilla (optic disc) is the entry of the optic nerve and blood vessels. It is a blind spot, as it lacks light-sensitive receptor cells.

The retina is fastened tightly to the lower layer at the point of papilla of the optic nerve and anterior edge, but the remainder is attached only very loosely. Therefore, when the eyeball is cut along the equator, the retina comes off easily. Even when alive, retinal separation is not rare. Once the retina is separated from the lower layer, the detached part cannot take in sufficient nutrition, resulting in the loss of sight.

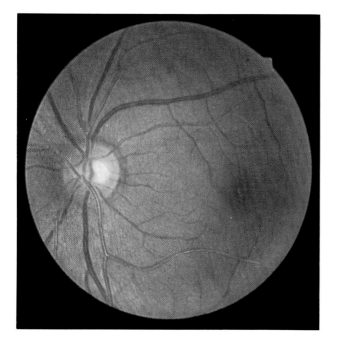

Normal fundus (in life)
By the courtesy of Dr. Masatoshi Fukuda, Department of Ophthalmology, University of Tokyo Branch Hospital, Tokyo.

CROSS-SECTIONS OF THE BODY (Female)

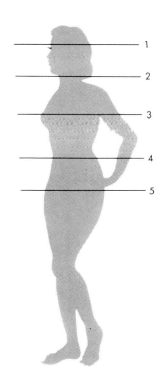

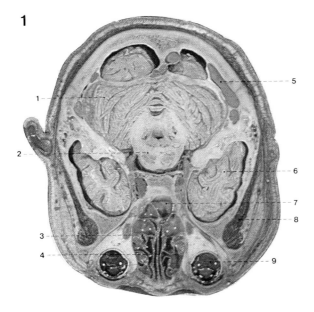

1

1. cerebellum
2. pons
3. ethmoid sinuses
4. septum of nose
5. transverse sinus
6. temporal lobe of the cerebrum
7. sphenoid sinus
8. temporalis m.
9. eyeball

2

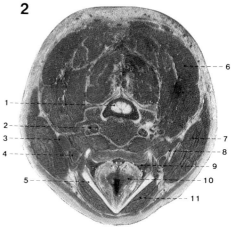

1. spinal cord
2. vertebral a. and v.
3. internal jugular vein
4. common carotid a.
5. thyroid cartilage
6. trapezius
7. sternocleidomastoid m.
8. vagus and hypoglossal n.
9. pharynx
10. laryngeal vestibule
11. sterno-, and thyrohyoid m.

3

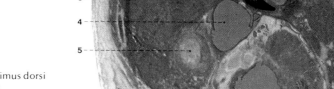

1. spinal cord
2. intervertebral disc
3. esophagus
4. inferior vena cava
5. diaphragm and liver
6. mammary gland
7. latissimus dorsi
8. aorta
9. lung
10. left ventricle
11. right ventricle
12. costal cartilage

4

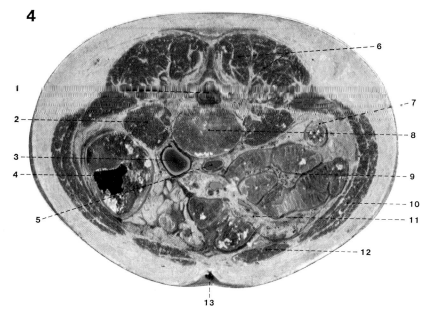

1. cauda equina
2. psoas major m.
3. inferior vena cava
4. cecum
5. aorta
6. longissimus and iliocostalis m.
7. descending colon
8. vertebra
9. small intestine
10. transversus, int. obliq., ext. obliq. abdominis
11. mesentery
12. rectus abdominis m.
13. navel

5

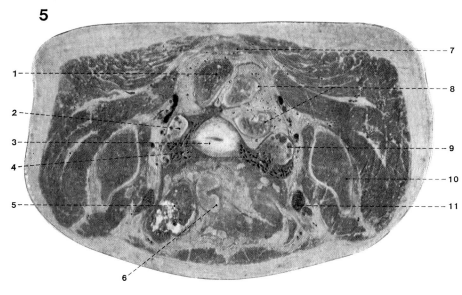

1. rectum
2. ovary
3. uterus
4. vena plexus
5. cecum
6. small intestine
7. sacrum
8. sigmoid colon
9. ovary
10. ilium
11. external iliac a. and v.